Dear Joseph, Love, Mom

S.H. Harlow

ISBN 978-1-64299-838-2 (paperback)
ISBN 978-1-64299-884-9 (hardcover)
ISBN 978-1-64299-839-9 (digital)

Copyright © 2018 by S.H. Harlow

All rights reserved. No part of this publication may be reproduced, distributed, or transmitted in any form or by any means, including photocopying, recording, or other electronic or mechanical methods without the prior written permission of the publisher. For permission requests, solicit the publisher via the address below.

Christian Faith Publishing, Inc.
832 Park Avenue
Meadville, PA 16335
www.christianfaithpublishing.com

Printed in the United States of America

This is a book about love, bravery, strength of spirit, and the discrimination faced by the disabled on a daily basis. It is my family's story, but it is a story surely shared by the disabled and their families throughout the world.

This book is dedicated to my son, Joseph, and also to all disabled people and their families throughout the world. My hope is that by reading this book, by getting to know one family's experience in navigating the world of the disabled, the world will finally recognize the attributes of the disabled and the value of their existence in this world. The disabled display an incredible amount of bravery on a daily basis and, for the most part, display no malice towards others. They are therefore a segment of the population that should be emulated and not discriminated against. The world could be a much better place if people became able to see and understand these attributes and treat the disabled with the dignity and respect that they earn every day of their lives just by being themselves.

Dear Joseph,

I have been trying to write this letter to you for a very long time but haven't been able to organize my thoughts and have found myself struggling to find the right words to convey those thoughts to you ... and there is so much that I want, and need, to say.

First, of course, I want to tell you how much I love you. I started to fall in love with you the second that I found out that you were going to be a part of my life, and I know that I will still be loving you after I take my final breath. I never knew that such a love existed. The intensity of that love took me by surprise. It is such an overwhelming, all-encompassing, all-consuming feeling that I don't think that there are any words to adequately describe it.

Your love has changed me. You have changed me. I don't remember who I was before I had you, but I am sure that I am not that same person. I don't know who I would be today if not "Joseph's mom," but I know that I can never be anyone else again. Being your mother was how I came to define, even identify, myself. You were my world.

I believe that you came here to complete my education, to help me see what I had not previously seen, and, along the way, assist others in learning those things that they needed to learn to complete their education. I know that I was not always the most willing student, but you were the kind of teacher that students love to hate. You were unbending in your methods, and I sometimes felt that I was fighting for my very existence, that the part of "me" that was "me" was fighting to survive. I sometimes felt like I was drowning. I do realize, though, that you were tough on me because you believed in me. I sometimes wish that you hadn't believed so strongly in me, but I realize that is who you were and who I needed you to be.

You Taught Me about Unconditional Love

The most important thing that you taught me about was unconditional love. There is no other place that I could have learned this. The parent-child relationship is the only relationship that exists between human beings where this kind of love exists. All other forms of love demand something from the individuals involved. There are always conditions attached to obtaining and keeping other forms of love. You loved me just for being me. I didn't have to be beautiful or sexy, smart or witty, rich or accomplished, of the "right" religion or the "right" color. You allowed me to just be me. Do you have any idea how refreshing, how uncomplicated and easy that was … that I didn't have to pretend to be something that I might not innately be, that what I was was enough? You are the love of my life, and although I know that I was undeserving of it, I thank you for this gift of unconditional love that you always gave me. I was given that unique opportunity to see with my heart, a vision much more enlightened and clear than any of my other senses could ever offer me. This unconditional love was the basis for everything else that you taught me, so it is only fitting that this should have been my first lesson.

You Taught Me about the Little Things in Life

You taught me that those "little" things in life that most people take for granted are the things that make life worth living. I remember listening to other children laughing and looking forward to the day when I would hear that sound spill from you. And when I finally did first hear you laugh, I knew the thrill that the great composers must have felt when first hearing the sounds of their masterpieces. You are *my* masterpiece. Your laugh could bring me from zero to sixty in a split second! I experienced a lightness in my soul and a burst of joy in my heart when I heard the purity of that sound emanating from your little body. Your laugh was honest and full of delight. It inspired a feeling of pure joy and a lightness of the soul and, if only for a moment, helped people to forget themselves and willingly plunge into that pool of delight that you created just by being you. Your laugh brightened my day and infused me with strength. It was intoxicating!

I lived to see you smile. Your smile was my light in the darkness. It was the one thing that could dispel that darkness that I felt in my very soul when I watched you suffer day after day. I knew that if you could smile through the dark days that you experienced, I had no right to allow that shroud of darkness to descend over me for any length of time. And I would do anything to make you smile no matter how silly it made me appear, for to make you happy was one of the most important missions in my life. I was called names and belittled because of the foolishness I employed in bringing a smile to your beautiful face, but I just chalked it up to other people's ignorance. They didn't know you or me. They didn't understand what your life was like and, therefore, couldn't possibly understand my need to attempt to extract as much joy from this existence for you as I could.

Ever since you were a baby, as soon as I knew that you were awake, I would charge up the stairs, making as much noise as possible to let you know that I was on my way, and then burst into the room where you were sleeping. Your little neck would be twisted around, watching me come through the bedroom door, a smile extending from ear to ear, your face lit up with happiness. I would run over to you and say, "My Joseph, my Joseph is up? I have been missing you!" I would then grab you up and crush your little body to mine, planting kisses all over your beautiful face, telling you over and over again how much I had missed you and how much I loved you. You would throw your little arms around my neck and squeeze me to you, giggling all the while, kicking your chubby little legs in excitement, basking in the warmth of a love that you had always been sure was yours without conditions.

We would then get on my bed and hug, kiss, and "talk." I could never resist putting my nose to the nape of your neck and smelling you. I swear that I could have picked you out of any baby put before me just by your smell! Daddy would join us if he wasn't working, but more often than not, it was just you and me, kid. We also got together on the bed before you went to sleep at night. We began and ended each day together this way so that you would always feel secure in the fact that you had a mommy and a daddy who loved you and couldn't wait until we got to be awake together again!

For as long as I can remember, when we would drive by the water treatment plant and high school by the side of the highway, a smile would explode across your face. You would start giggling uncontrollably and would kick your feet. You seemed to be bursting with joy! There was, to Daddy and me, nothing special about this particular stretch of highway, but you reacted the same way each time we passed by this spot. You had the same reaction when we drove into the development where we lived.

There were other times when I would observe you smiling for no obvious reason. I would go into your room at night to check on you after I had put you to bed. You would be smiling from ear to ear and "talking" while staring at a particular corner of the ceiling. I could not see whatever it was that you were seeing, but you would look at me and direct my eyes to that particular part of the ceiling, wanting to share the joy of whatever it was that you were seeing.

When you were little, we would go to a large store that had a huge fan blowing, I imagine to keep the hot air out in the summer months. You would laugh so hard when I pushed you through it, and your body would actually be trembling with excitement. I would do this a few times just to make you laugh. You also got a kick out of being pushed out the door of the administrative office of this store. I would say, "One … two … three," and then push you quickly through the door. This made you positively giddy! So … I would do this a number of times because you enjoyed it so much. Daddy told me one time that a man had come up to him and told him that the man in line behind him had said, "What is wrong with that kid?" The man then pointed to Daddy and said, "That is his father. Why don't you ask him?" I do not know what it was about these seemingly inconsequential things that brought you such joy, but you had that ability to find joy in the simplest moments. I don't remember when it was that you stopped finding this activity joyful, but I know how sad it made me feel that something had been lost, and try as I might, I could not make you laugh at this anymore.

I will always wish that I could have known those unseeable and unknowable things that made you smile and laugh. I have always been one of those people who need to know the why of things, but I am beginning to realize that I will just have to be satisfied with knowing that there are things that I will never understand and that I will just have be satisfied with the knowledge that these unknown things brought you joy.

Your hugs helped to ground me. You presented me with a variety of hugs. There was that backwards hug that you gave when sitting next to me in the chair where you would reach your arm around the front of my neck and pull my head to yours. There was the hug where you would take my hand and place it against your cheek. There was the hug where you simply laid your head against me. There was, more recently, the hug where you just touched me with your hand. And finally, there was the hug that I liked best … the hug where you would throw your little arms around me and squeeze me tight. When your little arms were around me, I felt as if I was infused with the strength of Goliath. I believed that I could face anything that life threw my way, although surely not entirely as gracefully as you, but I was still the student.

Your kisses were a seal of your love, proof of the absolute goodness and sweetness encased in that little body of yours. They were whispers from your very soul that I was a worthy recipient of your love, and when I felt your beautiful, slobbery little lips against my cheek, I understood this. I always needed those kisses no matter how messy or caveman-like your presentation.

I am not sure that I can properly describe the feeling that suffused my body when you put your little hand in mine. It spoke to me of trust and was further proof of your unconditional love for me. A feeling of peace and serenity descended over me. It made me feel like I was home.

Your smile, your laughter, your hugs, your kisses, your touch … all of these "little" things that cost me absolutely nothing infused me with a sense of strength and completeness. They were the medicines that kept me going, and I was addicted to them.

You Taught Me to Trust My Instincts

You taught me to trust my instincts, my senses, and my "gut." I have always been told to trust my gut instincts because they are generally right, but this is something that is easier said than done. We tend to question ourselves, especially when in a situation where our decisions could have very dire consequences. This I have always known, and yet early on, I felt that I should trust those people who were supposed to be experts in their fields.

Everyone seems to want to give the new mother advice on how to take care of their child. One thing that almost everyone told me was to not pick you up every time you cried. They told me that if I did, I would spoil you. I never listened to them. It was my opinion that when you cried, you were crying for a reason, and there was no way that I was going to ignore this. You were never one to cry without reason. In fact, you never cried at those times when anyone else on the face of the planet would have been screaming in agony.

There was one time when you were outside playing in your Flintstone car. I had just put socks on you because they were thick, and I felt that they would protect your feet. I was wrong, and you suffered because of my bad judgment. You liked to go up to the top of one of the neighbors' driveways because it had a steeper pitch than the rest of the driveways in the cul-de-sac, and you would then go down it as fast as you could. You would drag your feet on the ground, though, and by the time you stopped, you had scraped most of the skin off the sides of your big toe. I was horrified when I saw this, but you didn't seem to even notice that you were hurt. You didn't begin to cry until I started to clean and disinfect your toe!

I had ignored that voice inside of me that had told me to put shoes on your feet and you had hurt yourself. This, as well as everything else that you ever showed me, was only proof that I was right to trust my gut and that, when you did cry, pick you up and comfort you. I think that it made you feel supremely safe and secure in the fact that you were loved and that when you called for help, help would always come and you would not be alone. This was just one more confirmation that I should listen to myself where you were concerned and to also listen and look for any and all signs that you might send my way.

You began to reject my hugs when you were between one and two years of age. You would throw yourself away from me when I would pull your little body to mine. I almost dropped you when you first started doing this but quickly learned to tighten my hold on you when I felt you start to pull away. I didn't understand why you did this at first, although I remember feeling a tingling sensation in my spine and a crushing fear in my heart as I considered what might be going on. You no longer wanted me to play with you, choosing to do your own thing. It was at this same time that I noticed that you were not looking into my eyes. I remember feeling fear in the pit of my stomach as I began to consider that you might be autistic. My heart and mind hadn't wanted to accept the fact that you might have autism, so I had pushed that thought aside, trying to find any other reason for your behavior. When your doctor said that she didn't think that you had autism, I chose to believe her because the alternative was unthinkable to me. So even though my gut had told me what the truth was, my heart would not allow me to accept it. I later found out that these "feelings" that I had had been right when you were diagnosed with autism.

I always knew when you were getting sick because I could smell the sweetness of the mucous in your throat. I knew that within days, your temperature would be climbing towards that 105-degree mark. I knew that I would be looking at a full week without sleep as Daddy and I struggled to keep your temperature as close to normal as we could. I knew this well in advance of your doctor being able to detect anything with tests, and the tests were apparently mandatory, but I was powerless to prevent the inevitable fever from ravaging your tiny body.

I knew when your temperature was rising before anyone else could detect it because I knew how you felt when you were well. A simple touch could alert me that your body heat was rising because I knew you. I knew how you felt, how you smelled, how you sounded, how you looked, and how you acted. I did not need a thermometer to tell me this, only to tell me how high your temperature was.

I knew when looking into your beautiful eyes if there was less than that brilliant sparkle, that your little body was not feeling well, and that I had better keep my guard up and watch for signals that I knew you would give me that your situation was going downhill.

I knew when a bad seizure was about to come on because you taught me the signals to look for. The signals changed as your condition changed, so I had to be constantly on the lookout for new signs. It is amazing what the subconscious mind picks up and stores for use later on.

I remember when you had your first grand mal seizure. You were sick again, but I sensed that something was different this time. I always slept on a mattress next to your bed when you were sick so that I could get to you quickly and keep watch on you throughout the night. My very being seemed to be on edge this particular night. I felt a tingling sensation and thought that the hair was actually standing up on the back of my neck. I had no idea what was coming down the pike but sensed that whatever was coming was going to be bad. You had been vomiting throughout the evening. By the fourth time, this had turned to dry heaves, as you had nothing left in your stomach. I heard a change in your breathing and kept getting up to check on you, even though you were hooked up to the pulse oximeter, which was telling me that you were breathing fine. I even called the doctor, telling her that something was wrong with you.

And then all hell broke loose at about one in the morning. Your pulse oximeter went off, and I sprang into action. Your lips were blue, so I tried to give you oxygen but couldn't get the machine to work. I began muttering to myself and begging God to help me. That didn't help either, so I picked you up and ran downstairs to get another oxygen tank but still couldn't get you to pink up, so I called 911. You came around just before they walked in the door, so I felt foolish for having panicked. I almost sent them away, but you went back into another seizure, so we went off to the hospital. This incident, probably more than any other, taught me to trust my instincts, that if my "gut" was sending me a warning, I needed to listen.

You had the same symptoms a few months later. You had tried to grab onto me while I was loading your things into the car to take you to Easter Seals. When you landed, you had hit the front of your head on the carpet. I had picked you up to comfort you and make sure that you were all right. You had stopped crying and seemed fine, so we left to get you to school. I honestly thought that you were okay. I dropped you off and then went to pick up my work, but I felt uneasy, so I stopped back by the school to make sure that you were okay. As soon as I entered your classroom, the teacher and aides ran up to me and said that they had been trying to contact me. We didn't have cell phones at that time, but got them after this incident so that we would be able to be reached at any time anywhere. They told me that you had been throwing up since shortly after I had dropped you off. My thoughts immediately went back to that night a few months earlier. I got you into the car and headed back home.

I felt frantic the entire time I had you in the car, looking back at you every couple of minutes. One time, I sensed that you were going to vomit again, so I pulled off the road and got you out of the car so that you could vomit on the side of the road. No one stopped to help. When I felt that you were done, I got you back into the car and got home as quickly as I could. I called Daddy as soon as we got home to see where he was and to tell him that we needed to get you to the doctor. I was afraid that you were going to go into a bad seizure and knew that I could not drive and take care of you at the same time. He got back to the house within fifteen minutes, and we headed to the doctor's office.

It was not long after we got there that you started vomiting again. The doctor immediately took you into a room and started to examine you. I was holding you while she was looking you over. I saw your eyes roll back and said, "He's having a seizure." Daddy and the doctor looked at your pulse oximeter and, since it was showing a normal reading, said, "No, you weren't." I then said, "I don't care what that machine is saying, I have seen this before!" And then your numbers started dropping. Your jaw started to clench. I noticed that your tongue was sticking out, so I put my fingers between your teeth to prevent you from biting it off, while the doctor got a tongue depressor. I know now that I could have had my fingers bitten off, but all I could think at that time was to save your tongue. We called 911 and went off to the hospital.

You started having ear infections when you were four months old, so you were put on antibiotics. The thing is, the ear infections didn't go away for five months. I wanted to take you to have tubes put in your ears, but I was the only one who felt this necessary. I remember, one night, you started screaming, and no matter what I did, I could not console you. Honey, I just couldn't figure out what was wrong or how to make it better. You stopped screaming after about half an hour, and I then noticed fluid coming out of your ear. Your eardrum had burst. I didn't know. I am so sorry, but everything with you was a learning experience, and I didn't possess the pertinent knowledge until after the fact. I can only imagine the pain that you were experiencing, but I will always feel pain in my heart that I wasn't more proactive in preventing your suffering. Tubes were finally placed in your ears. I never, after this, let anyone, regardless of how many letters they had following their name, ever dissuade me from taking the action that I felt necessary to prevent something like this from happening again.

Your ENT doctor later told us that you had been hearing as if listening to someone while under water. I think that this increased your ability to concentrate because you had to listen so much harder to hear everything than the average person. I remember one time when you were cruising around the living room in your walker and heard one of your stories being read by someone on the television. You stopped what you were doing, went over to the TV, listened until the story was over, and then went on your way.

You also had lazy eyes, so you were fighting to interact with the world with deficiencies in two of your major senses. When I think of

DEAR JOSEPH, LOVE, MOM

how hard you had to work to hear and see the things in your world, how hard you had to struggle to maneuver around your world, I am always awestruck at the magnitude of strength and perseverance that you never failed to exhibit.

You Taught Me about Fear

Everyone feels fear, I know, but I don't think that most people are as intimately acquainted with fear as you taught me to be. I don't believe that I have lived one day of my life since your birth without fear being an unwelcome companion, threatening to cut off my breathing as it swelled in my throat. This fear, though, kept all of my senses heightened, on alert. I was constantly listening, watching, smelling, and touching, knowing that your life depended on my being able to quickly sense any abnormalities in these things. I suppose fear has been something that was necessary for your survival, for it kept me on my toes, keeping that fight-or-flight reaction ready to kick in at a moment's notice.

We didn't know if you were going to live or die when you were first born. You were in distress, and they had to take you. Your tiny little body had begun to fail, organ by organ, within hours of your birth. I didn't know this, though, as I had been given something to knock me out after being shown you. You were the most beautiful child that I had ever seen!

I remember waking up after you had been taken and seeing Daddy. He looked like he had been crying, but denied this when I asked him. When he finally told me the truth, the only thing that I could think of was getting to you. They wouldn't let me go to you right away, though, because I had had a C-section and wasn't allowed to move for twelve hours. I finally got to see you at one o'clock in the morning. You were lying on your stomach, hooked up to all kinds of machines with tubes coming out of every orifice, and it sounded as if the very act of breathing was causing you excruciating pain. Your little hands and feet were black. We were advised that if they didn't pink up, you might lose them. I had never felt so helpless in my life, a feeling that I was to repeatedly re-experience throughout your lifetime. All I could do was stand there, with tears running down my face, feeling like my heart was being ripped out of my chest.

That was the only time that I was allowed to touch you for the next thirteen days. I touched your little hind end, and it was so soft that it felt like I was touching air. I took your little hand in mine and you curled your tiny little fingers around my fingers. Your little fingers were so cold!

You were then put on what they called "zero" stimulation, and we weren't allowed any physical contact with you. We even had a priest come in and give you last rites because it was looking like you were not going to make it. I was so afraid that I would never get to hold your little body next to mine while you were still alive. Within days, your body became swollen with fluid. You looked like the Pillsbury Doughboy!

What joy I experienced when I finally did get to hold you! I was scared to death, but I guess that is what is meant by an experience being bittersweet. The skin on your face was sagging because you had been so swollen, but to me you were still the most beautiful child in the world and I never wanted to release you from my arms again.

It was on the thirteenth day of your life that you were given your first real food. I got to give you your first bottle of formula. You sucked that bottle down so fast that everyone who witnessed it was amazed! You never looked back after that first bottle. It was as if you were saying, "As God is my witness, I will never be hungry again." You became a definite lifelong foodie after that day. It always amazed people, the amount of food that you could consume. You never got fat though, but you were definitely solid. People would go to pick you up and be surprised at how heavy you actually were, deceived by your very fit-looking body.

I think that we came really close to losing you again on your first Thanksgiving Day. We had just finished preparing our Thanksgiving dinner and headed up the stairs to get showered. I was bouncing you over my shoulder because this always made you laugh, but this time when I laid you down on the bed, you had the strangest look on your face. Your face was expressionless and your eyes looked distant. I hadn't seen that look before and was trying to figure out what it meant when I noticed that your lips were turning blue. My first thought was that you were choking on something, so I turned you over and started pounding on your back. I yelled to Daddy to come quickly, that something was wrong, but you appeared better by the time that he got there. You looked tired the rest of the day and later on started vomiting, so we ended up taking you to the hospital, where you were admitted.

It was a good thing that we decided to take you to the hospital because the next morning at six o'clock, while I was giving you your bottle, it happened again. You had that same empty stare, and your lips had turned blue. I was petrified! All I could think to do was to scream for the nurse. I didn't think, at that time, as my mind had shut off, to consider that there were other children and parents in the room. All I knew was that you were not breathing and I needed to get help to you right away. I tried to call Daddy after the nurse took you, but I couldn't think. My mind was blank. I ended up calling the wrong number and waking up some poor man. I then asked the nurse to call Daddy because I could not pull our phone number out of my brain.

They couldn't figure out what was wrong with you, so we were sent home a few days later, only to return again within two days with the same symptoms. They ended up sending us to the nearest children's hospital, but they, after extensive testing, couldn't figure out what was going on either, so we were again sent home ... only to return the next day with the same symptoms.

While we were in the emergency room, we tried to explain to them that you were having cycles of these symptoms. We told them that when they happened, you had three episodes over a period of an hour and that they needed to hook you up to the EEG right away if they wanted to catch anything, as you had already had two of the episodes. They didn't listen to us, and just as we had said would happen, you had another "episode" before you were hooked up to the EEG machine. You didn't have any further symptoms for another five days. It was then that you were given the diagnosis of epilepsy. We now, at least, had an idea of what we were facing. We were instructed on, and given, equipment to monitor your breathing and alert us to when a seizure was occurring.

We never had complete control of your seizures, but learned to read the signs of an impending attack. They were always worse when you were sick. There was one day when you were running a high fever when you had sixteen seizures within an hour. I was trying to work, plus keep you hydrated and cool. Your body was like a little steam oven and you refused to let me give you any fluids. I was tired and relatively new to this whole "parent thing" but got smarter as time went on. I found that I could force fluids on you with a syringe, directing the fluid towards your cheek. I finally had to admit defeat that day though, called the doctor, and brought you to the hospital.

I was again reminded to trust my instincts with regard to my observations when members of the hospital staff almost killed you when you were about one and a half years old. You were, again, in the hospital with a high fever, as you had been about one week of every month of your life. This particular time, when they brought your medication, I noticed that it was only a fraction of what you generally took. I mentioned this to them and was told, "This is a really concentrated form of this medication, so he doesn't need to take as much." I remember being surprised and wondering why your doctor would make you take such a larger dose of a less concentrated medication. I made a mental note to call the doctor when we got out of the hospital and ask if he could prescribe you the medication that the hospital had given you. I thought it weird that your doctor would not know about this medication.

It turned out that you *were* being given the concentrated form of the medication. We were informed that the pharmacist had thought that the dose of medication that was prescribed by your doctor was too high and, therefore, had cut the dose to one-twentieth of what you should be taking, so after a couple of doses, you basically had no medicine in your body.

I knew something was wrong later that night, because you kept moaning and would not go to sleep. As I held you, I felt your body jump and then stiffen up periodically. I called the nurse and told her what I had been seeing. I told her that you had been sleeping through the night without any problems since you were six weeks old. I questioned whether your medication levels had come back okay, but they just blew me off, saying that they were going to draw more levels at six in the morning. I called them to your room again shortly afterward and told them that something was very wrong. It was then that they decided to take some blood and do a drug level. They came back twenty minutes later, telling me that they had been unable to get blood to do a drug level.

Daddy had always taken you to get your blood drawn because I was generally working, but I also couldn't stand to see the look of betrayal in your eyes when I allowed anyone to hurt you by sticking a needle in your arm. I, therefore, didn't know that they could have done a finger-stick and gotten enough blood to do the drug levels. The nurses on duty that night should have known this though, but they did nothing, saying only that they would try again in a few hours.

A few hours proved to be too late. You went into an intractable seizure and all I could do was stand there, helplessly watching, while six adults held your little body down and tried to inject Ativan into your arm to stop the seizure. I just stood there in shock, tears streaming down my face, and when your doctor came in, I asked her, "How did this happen?" She told me that she had prescribed the correct dose of medication, but that the pharmacist had felt it was too much. She told me that they had drawn a drug level at about eight in the evening and it had shown that your levels were "ridiculously" low. They felt that, because you had been being given your medication, the lab had "blown" the test. I then asked her whether it would not have been more appropriate to do the test again and make sure that it was correct than to not do it and assume that the test had been blown.

During that same admission, they had also not paid enough attention to your IV. It had gone bad and the fluid had built up in your little hand and lower arm, until they were so swollen that the skin over these areas died and we had to peel it off!

It was decided that you needed to be airlifted to the children's hospital. I left to drive to the other hospital while they got the paperwork finished. I made it there before the helicopter did!

We incorrectly assumed that you would be better taken care of there, since it was a world-renowned children's hospital, when we were unable to be with you, but again, we were wrong. One day, when we got there, another parent, whose child was in the same room with you, came up to us and said that the nurse who had been taking care of you had "freaked out" when you had one of your seizures and another nurse had to intervene.

During your stay there, we found that the nurses were unwilling to listen to any advice from the parents. I assume that they felt that their medical training made their care superior to that of the children's parents. I walked in one day when a nurse was giving you your medicine. I had told them that they needed to mix a couple of ounces of formula with your phenobarbital because it was extremely hot/spicy and you would choke on it. They gave it to you straight, anyway, and just as they had been told you would do, you started choking and gagging, doing so for twenty minutes. I was furious! They were more willing to listen to me after that. We never dared to leave you in a hospital unattended after this. We decided it was necessary for one of us to be with you at all times so that you would be given the correct dosages of your medications and that your medications would be administered in the way that we knew you would be able to tolerate. It was a good thing that we made this decision because we witnessed numerous potential mistakes which were averted because we were there to prevent them from happening.

Honey, I was afraid every second of every minute of every hour of every day of your life, fearing that I wasn't going to be able to do the right thing at the right time to save you. I had no choice but to swallow that fear and keep trying ... to never give up ... to stand up for you (and myself) and fight for what I knew was right, for what my gut was telling me was right, because I knew that that was exactly what you would do. Your whole life was a testament to not giving up, so how could I?

My very worst day, the day that I am surprised fear did not actually suffocate me, my personal 9/11, was October 15, 2001. You had been sick for five days, with a fever approaching 105 degrees. We had been alternating Tylenol and Motrin every two hours to keep your fever down, as well as giving you tepid baths in between doses of these medications. Your temperature had finally been normal for twenty-four hours, so I decided to start to cut back on the medicine to every four hours. Daddy had just left for work, and as seemed to always be the case, all hell broke loose.

Your little body started to tremble violently, so I knew that your temperature was skyrocketing. When I took your temperature, you were already at 103 degrees, having risen over four degrees within fifteen minutes time. I gave you Motrin, then picked you up and ran upstairs to get you into the bathtub. You were shaking and crying and clinging to me. I was trying to pour water over you, hold you, and calm you simultaneously. Your eyes then rolled up in your head and you started to turn blue. I picked you up and ran down the hall to the bedroom where we kept your medicine and oxygen.

I inserted the Diastat in your butt and placed the cannula in your nose. It wasn't working. The doctor had always told us to smack you on the back to stimulate your breathing, so I tried that, but you wouldn't come back to me. Your lips and nail beds were black at this point. I could feel panic ripping through my body. I raced to the phone and dialed 911. I could feel my whole body shaking and the muscles in my throat starting to tighten. My eyes were burning as I fought back tears. I was frantic! I knew I had to try to calm myself down, so I began mumbling to myself, not knowing what else to do. I knew that I had to quell the panic that I was experiencing so that I could communicate effectively with the people at the 911 center and continue working on you, but I was beginning to feel like I couldn't breathe. I could feel myself starting to fall apart from the inside out. I kept working on you throughout this time, but could feel the fear continuing to escalate inside me, as nothing that I did to bring you back was working.

And then you went still. Your lips and nail beds were black. Your eyes were fixed in an empty stare. I put my ear to your chest and could not hear your heartbeat. I tried to find a pulse in your neck and at your wrist but could not. I put my face to your nose and mouth and could feel no air movement. That is when I lost it. I started crying and said, "He's not breathing. I can't get him breathing." I must have scared the 911 operator because another person came on the phone. She tried to calm me by telling me that an ambulance was on the way and attempting to engage me in conversation to keep me calm, but I wouldn't be calmed. The only thing that I could think to do at that point was to scream out, "Please, God, no!" I hit you on the back, as I had been instructed to do by your neurologist. You immediately started coughing and came back to me. I started kissing you and laughing, not immediately picking you up because your lips were still blue and you, therefore, needed to continue on the oxygen. The ambulance then arrived and you were taken to the hospital.

You, Daddy, and I went through a lot of harrowing days, but this is the one day, the one memory, that never fails to reduce me to a sobbing, blithering idiot. It is the one memory that is still as painful today as it was when it happened.

You were placed on what we called a "miracle" drug when you were five years old. This medicine brought your seizures down from twenty minutes to thirty seconds! That was the good aspect of the drug. The bad aspect was that you would have what Daddy and I called "screaming" seizures. You would get a look of absolute terror in your eyes and then utter a blood-curdling scream. The sound of that scream cut through me to my very soul. I actually felt pain in my chest and felt my throat constricting.

You always knew when a seizure was coming on and, if you were able, would try to get to Daddy or me. With these particular seizures, you would get a sort of crazed look in your eyes, like something was scaring you to death, and then begin looking frantically around for someone to "save" you from whatever it was that was tormenting you. There were times when I did not have you in my line of vision, and when I heard you scream, I would drop whatever I was doing and run to you as fast as my legs would go.

There was one time that I was upstairs putting away laundry while you were downstairs watching one of your videos. I heard that scream, dropped the laundry basket, and started running. I looked over the balcony and saw you frantically making your way towards the kitchen, where you thought I was. I considered jumping over the balcony because I figured that I would be able to get to you sooner but, when I spent another second thinking about this, I knew that was more dangerous than smart. I raced down the stairs and reached you as you were coming out of the living room. You ran to me and put your arms around my neck until the seizure was over, having been soothed by my comforting words and loving embrace.

When these seizures would happen, the only thing that I could do was hold you close to me and tell you over and over again, "I've got you. I've got you. It's okay. I love you." That seemed to be enough to get you through the seizure, and you would then go back to whatever it was that you were doing before the onset of the seizure, leaving me to try to collect myself and slow my heartbeat to a normal rhythm.

Every time that you had a seizure, and this was often, I was nearly paralyzed with fear no matter what type of seizure it was. It took every ounce of my strength to keep working through the fear. I, at times, felt that I had no reserves left to call upon but somehow found some small measure of strength. I sometimes felt so totally drained following particularly bad seizures that I pretty much just collapsed onto the couch after making sure that you are okay and safe.

I started to climb into bed with you every night after you had fallen asleep, after that first bad seizure when you were nine months old. I did this up until the time of your last hospitalization, when I could no longer fit in the hospital bed with you. I curled up next to you and put my ear to your chest or back and listened. I listened to the rhythmic beating of your heart in your chest. I listened to the sound of air rushing into and out of your lungs. These sounds were so soothing to me. They were music to my very soul. They assured me that life still inhabited your body. I realized that you were hooked up to a machine that will let me know if you were not breathing properly, but I needed to hear those things for myself with my own ears. I learned that machines cannot tell the whole story. I needed to personally hear your heart beating and the air moving through your lungs to feel true comfort in my heart and mind, always acutely aware that this music could be easily taken away.

I sometimes lay in bed with you for hours, sometimes falling asleep next to you. You looked so peaceful when you were sleeping. You were free from agitation, frustration, sadness, pain, and anger.

I would look at your beautiful face, with your thick lashes, full eyebrows, chubby cheeks, elegant nose, perfectly shaped lips, and beautiful, thick head of hair. I would look at your elegant hands, with your long, pianist fingers. I would look at your beautiful feet, with your little toes lined up like peas in a pod. I would look at your long torso and long, chubby legs. It was as if I was trying to sear these images, these memories, into my brain so that I would never forget, so that, should something happen to you, I would have these pictures forever in my head to remind me of how lucky I once was to have you in my life. I sometimes wonder if you could feel me looking at you as you lay there sleeping.

I remember the fear that I had felt when I first began to suspect that you had autism. Your eye contact had become basically nonexistent. You kept throwing yourself away from me and wanted to be by yourself. I mentioned these things to your doctor, but she assured me that you were not autistic. I chose to believe her and not listen to my gut because I was too much of a coward. I chose not to listen to her because of the fear that the word "autism" inspired in the depths of my soul. I didn't want to believe that you would be forced to climb that particular mountain when you had already been forced to scale so many other mountains in your short time on this earth. But what was appropriately said in the movie *City of Angels*, "Some things are true, whether you believe them or not."

The more I learned about autism, the angrier I got. When we were finally able to afford to chelate you—and the level of mercury in your body was off the charts with your aluminum level not far behind—I felt an anger that I had never experienced before. I also felt let down by my government for having allowed those poisons to be put in the shots that I had been forced to give to you.

When you were about eight years old, you started to have bouts of pneumonia. As you got older, you started to develop it more often and it seemed to become more severe. There were times when the doctors did not seem to think that they would be able to save you. Daddy never told me that the doctors had said this, just as he had not told me that you were not expected to live much past the age of thirteen.

When we heard a change in your breathing, we would immediately check your oxygen levels, because we never knew if you were just sick or developing pneumonia. I got so scared when I saw your sats drop and knew that you did indeed have pneumonia and we would have to take you to the hospital. I got even more scared seeing you hooked up to all kinds of equipment to help you breathe, fearing that that time was the time that you were not going to be able to fight your way through it. You always seemed to bounce back, though, even through the worst cases of pneumonia. These were the moments that I prayed for, when my heart could stop feeling so tight with fear, and we could go home and resume our lives. Your lungs became damaged over the years from the repeated pneumonias and your last bout of pneumonia was your last bout of pneumonia. Your lungs were just too scarred to come back from this, and my worst fear was finally realized. I lost you.

You Taught Me to Sometimes Be Afraid of You

Honey, you also taught me to sometimes be afraid of you. You started having periods of unprovoked rage when you were about three. You would dig, bite, and/or pull my hair. It was never clear what brought these periods of rage on, but when these episodes began, you seemed to go so deeply into them that there was no changing course until the rage was exhausted.

Most times, the only thing that I could do was to run away from you, since trying to restrain you only made you angrier. You sometimes got up and ran after me, still very deeply in the throes of your rage. I can remember pulling anything large that I could into your path to slow you down so that I could get away. A couple of times, I even had to box myself into a corner, where you could not reach me, until your anger subsided.

There were times when you went into these rages when I was unable to distance myself from you, like when I had you on the toilet. I had to stay close to you so that I could catch you in case you had a seizure so that you would not slam your head against anything. I was also in harm's way when I had to feed you or give you a drink. You were in control at these times, knowing that I would not walk away, and you would come at me again and again.

When you were deep in this "Dr. Jekyll/Mr. Hyde" mode, I think that I actually felt like I did not like you very much. I found myself wishing for it to be over. I couldn't stand to see you suffer day after day. I was tired of being afraid. I was tired of not knowing from moment to moment, day to day, when you were going to go into a rage and hurt me. But even as these thoughts were racing through my brain, I knew that I couldn't stand it if you died. I knew that that would be the end of me. I knew that what I actually wanted was for both of us to live, not merely exist. I wanted you to be able to have the kind of life that we all deserve to have. I wanted you to be able to do all the things that little boys find enjoyment in doing. I wanted you to have the opportunity to experience all of the things that little boys experience. I wanted you to be able to breathe more easily and live a life free of any more suffering. And so when you were at death's door, I could not let you pass through it. I could not imagine a life without you.

I had to keep telling myself that this rage that you experienced was something that you could not control. I have to tell you, though, that your attacks hurt me not only physically but also psychologically. My mind kept telling me that it was the autism or that you were not feeling well that was causing these intense episodes of rage, but the attacks still elicited a heartbreaking pain that no amount of reasoning could allay. Everything that Daddy and I did was for you. I have always loved you more deeply than I could ever have imagined loving anyone and every physical attack from you cut me to my very soul. I sometimes could not reconcile myself with the fact that what was going on was beyond your control, that you didn't really want to hurt me, and I sometimes spent hours trying to get over the attacks.

I was sometimes too tired to fight with you anymore after one of these episodes. I would put you in bed and walk away, slamming the bedroom door as I left. I needed you to realize that you had hurt me and that I wanted you to think about what you had done. You would sometimes lie awake, saying, "Mom, Mom, Mom." It tore at my heart to not run in and put my arms around you, but I needed to lick my own wounds before I could administer to your need to be forgiven, all the while knowing that you had little or no control over these outbursts. I would return a little while later, hug and kiss you, tell you that I loved you, and tell you that I knew that these periods of rage were not intentional.

You Taught Me to Be Strong

By teaching me to fight my way through my fears, to keep trying, no matter what, you taught me to be strong and, although I know that I will never be as strong as you were and prayed that I would never have to be. I know that this, too, was an extremely important lesson for me. I cannot honestly say that I was never hovering over that line of giving up. I am ashamed of that. My only defense is that I was so god-awful tired and scared. But you always seemed to pull me back across that line and convince me to pick myself up, dust myself off, and start all over again.

People mistakenly thought that you were my weakness, but in truth, you were my strength. There is no way that I could have watched you valiantly battle your way through the attacks on your body, never giving up, and not known in my very soul that I had no choice, that I could never give up on you because you would never give up on yourself or me. Even in your most trying times, you exhibited unparalleled strength and a compassion I have never seen anywhere else.

Your most outstanding attribute has always been your strength of spirit. If every human being had your strength of spirit, no one would ever feel small or ugly or inadequate. They would know that whatever they are is enough and that knowledge would set them free.

When your little body would descend into the unimaginable hell of a seizure, which would last anywhere from ten to twenty minutes, I would do what I had been instructed to do for you medically, and then all I could do was kiss your beautiful face over and over again, tell you repeatedly that I loved you, and beg you to come back to me. I could see you struggling to come back. I know that you could sense the fear and desperation in my voice because as soon as you came out of the seizure, you would put your little arm around my neck, give me a weak laugh, and "pat" me, trying to assure me that the worst was over and that you were going to be okay. Your first thought was always to console me, to start the healing process on my battered heart. This offered me some relief, but I still could not escape the knowledge that you were still in exquisite pain from the violent contractions that had assaulted every muscle in your body and that you were fighting nausea that had your little belly doing somersaults.

When I would tell your neurologist about this, he would just snicker and say that what I had described was impossible. He wasn't there, though, and hadn't seen what I had seen. His knowledge came primarily from medical books and journals and things that he had seen in the office and hospital. I have to assume that he had never seen anything similar to what I described and was therefore unwilling to give credence to the observations of one of these children's mothers. He failed to understand that life doesn't always follow the information found in textbooks. Each of our bodies are uniquely different in some way.

You would drift off to sleep for a couple of hours after having a seizure, occasionally waking up to vomit. When you did finally wake up after the seizure, you had put this experience behind you as demonstrated by that beautiful smile and joyful laugh of yours. It was almost as if you just took it in stride, that this was just a normal part of life, and were able to leave the past in the past. Even though I know that these experiences enabled me to bounce back more quickly than most would from unpleasant experiences and situations, it inevitably took me much longer than you to distance myself from the horror of these experiences. You have been, and always will be, my little bumble.

People approached Daddy and me often and said, "I don't know how you do it. I could never do what you do." Honey, you taught me that we never know what we can do until we are pushed to our limits, which is something that people don't often consciously do until they have no other choice. We are then forced to find the strength, the courage, the power, to push ourselves further than we thought that we were capable of. People, as a rule, tend to not like to step outside of that little box that they create for themselves. We all get to a point in our lives where we just want to slow down and settle into that comfortable rut that we find ourselves entrenched in. We don't like to step out of our comfort zones.

All those times that people saw me spring into action when you had a seizure, I have no doubt that their eyes were telling them that they were seeing someone being brave, but they were wrong, at least as it related to me. They could not see that I was in tatters on the inside. They couldn't see that on the inside, my mind and body were screaming for help. They couldn't see the coward that actually stood, or knelt, at your side.

They didn't know how often I had wanted to run away from the excruciating pain that I felt every day of my life as I watched you suffer. They could not possibly have realized how I wanted to be freed from the gut-wrenching fear that had become my constant companion. And maybe they could not understand that I just could not just run away. My love for you forced me to stay. My love for you made me feel ashamed that I would ever even consider doing such a thing. My love made me feel a coward in your presence. How could I possibly leave you when I know that you would never leave me. How could I fail to try to emulate the unwavering courage that you exhibited every day of your life? You never let anything steal your joy away from you. You never lost your smile no matter what you went through, whether it be a seizure, just not feeling well, or verbal assaults on your person by people too close-minded to recognize the hero residing in your soul. So how could I not follow that life's tenet of "Pick yourself up, dust yourself off, and start all over again"?

So I donned this façade not for them but for you … always for you. I have never been brave. When your body was beating you up, I actually felt blows being dealt to my own body. When your little body was burning up with fever, I felt the flames lapping at my own flesh. All of my faux bravery was an illusion that I needed to present so that you would feel safe, so that you would feel that I had everything under control, so that you would not be afraid.

I never wanted you to feel afraid for one second longer than absolutely necessary. I tried to always be as close to you as I possibly could so that should a seizure start, those seconds that you were experiencing terror would not add up while I tried to get to you. I needed to get you into my arms to quell that fear that you were experiencing and to calm you with the sound of my voice and the warmth of my arms, assuring you that everything was going to be all right, knowing all the while that I was lying to you, that probability and statistics would say that nothing was ever going to be okay. I always knew in my very soul that you needed that illusion but am also aware that you alone could see through that illusion. I knew that you could hear the terror in my voice as I begged you to come back to me but also recognized my valiant attempt at bravery and, therefore, kept this knowledge to yourself.

You never let me develop a comfort zone. It seems that as soon as I figured out your signals, you changed them. I barely got a chance to take a breath and you were moving me on up the ladder. I somehow understand that this kind of training forced me to test my limits every day of my life. The simple act of getting you through every seizure, every illness, strengthened my reserves. You taught me to be strong. You showed me that I am much more capable than I ever dreamt I could be. You showed me that I could push my mind and body to its limits and then some.

I went days at a time with no sleep at all. I went years with so little sleep that my body acclimated and I was unable to sleep more than a few hours a night. I sometimes worked seventy-two-hour shifts in order to make enough money to keep a roof over our heads and keep our bills paid. I managed to work the equivalent of a couple of full-time jobs while also managing to take you to doctor's visits and therapy appointments and stay with you during your hospitalizations. I watched your little body beat itself up thousands of times. I knelt over your little body, blinded by tears, kissing your little face over and over again, telling you over and over again how much I loved you while begging you to come back to me. You faced each attack on your body with incredible strength and humility, but no matter how strong you may have made me, I know that I will never have the grace or strength that you possessed. And I always prayed that I would never need it. I have always been amazed at what your mind and body can go through and still survive. You were a model of strength that everyone should aspire to emulate.

You Taught Me to Stand Up and Fight

Every step of the way seemed to be a struggle, so I had to learn to stand up to people, even though I would much rather have been able to watch from the sidelines. This constant struggle was utterly exhausting! I have never liked arguments and often just turned away from confrontation. You taught me that no matter how uncomfortable it may be, we sometimes have to not cower at the prospect of a confrontation. Some things are worth fighting for and we have to find both the strength and courage within ourselves to stand up to the aggressors.

Daddy and I had quite a few heated discussions with members of the educational establishment. I always went into your classroom at different times to pick you up so that I could observe what was going on at different times of the day. I was appalled to notice that most times when I went in, they had you strapped into a car seat, shoved into a corner of the room, with nothing to do but twiddle your thumbs. They didn't think to provide you with a toy or book to keep you occupied. Their explanation was that they could not watch you and take care of the other children. It was then that we decided that you needed a one-on-one. But as with most situations such as this, we had to go up against the "bean counters" who always feel that if they turn down a request from a parent, the parents will just walk away and choose not to fight. They should really become more adept at recognizing those parents that *will* stand their ground and not give up when told no.

When we got an IEP scheduled to discuss the need for a one-on-one, this ended up being our main weapon. Daddy and I sat on one side of the table and the school had their army of employees on the other side of the table. They defended their opinion that there was no need for you to have someone assigned specifically to you because they felt that they were doing such a good job of attending to your needs. When I reminded the teacher that she had told me that they had to "restrain" you in a car seat because they couldn't watch you and take care of the other children, they were unable to defend their position. The teacher tried to deny that she had made this statement, but I backed her into a corner with her own words. She didn't like me very much after that.

I have to admit to there being a kind of freedom to not caring whether someone likes you or not. I never felt the need to back down from a confrontation with her when I felt that they were not acting in your best interests and possibly endangering your life.

One day, when I went into the classroom to pick you up, they were watching a movie and the room was pitch-black. I could hardly see my hand in front of my face. I found you and took you home. We had just walked through the door when you went into a bad seizure. All I could think was that had I picked you up even ten minutes later, this would have happened at school. They would not have been able to see your face, because the room was so dark, and you would have fallen to the floor, hitting your head. The next day, I told your teacher what had happened and conveyed my fear that had this happened at school, you would have been badly hurt. She seemed to take umbrage at my assessment, so I told them that they needed to have your face in view at all times so that they could catch any seizures before bodily harm was done.

It wasn't long after this incident that I went to pick you up and, again, had an issue with your care. I went into the classroom and was advised that you were outside playing in the courtyard. When I arrived in the courtyard, which was cement with a tiny patch of sand in the middle, I observed your one-on-one sitting on a bench at least a hundred feet from you, talking to another aide, while you walked around on this hard cement without your helmet on. I ran to you, picked you up, and then confronted this woman. I explained to her what you, and I, would face should you have a seizure and fall to the cement, smashing your head, while unprotected by your helmet, while she sat a hundred feet away leisurely having a conversation with a coworker. I told her that her job was basically to act as your "shadow." I went further to explain that a shadow, by its very definition, is basically an extension of something caused by backlighting, and would, therefore, require that she be in close proximity with you. I managed to make myself another enemy.

The final "nail in the coffin" with my relationship with your teacher came after we had taken you to see a specialist in autism. You had been given the diagnosis of autism and she, being a special education teacher, felt that this doctor's diagnosis was wrong. She felt that her assessment of you was the more correct diagnosis. She had, after all, gone to school to learn to teach ESE kids and also had two ESE children of her own. She told me that I should listen to the professionals, i.e. her. I was pretty sick of her superior attitude at this point, so I told her, "Where Joseph is concerned, I *am* the professional," picked you up, and turned and walked away.

Near the end of your time at this school, Easter Seals asked if they could do a story on you. We were, of course, very excited and told everyone about it. When the story was finally printed, we bought a bunch of papers so that we could send the story to friends and family. Your teacher, after reading the article, called the reporter and asked why her school had not been mentioned, stating that they worked very hard with you. The reporter attempted to explain to her that the story was actually on a past Easter Seals' student, but your teacher would have none of this and hung up on her.

I also had problems with your kindergarten teacher. She felt that you should not be in an autistic classroom. We explained to her that you had been diagnosed with autism, so you were exactly where you needed to be. We explained that you had been memorizing books since you were a few months old. Daddy and I always tried to tell your teachers and aides what you are interested in and what we had found worked best with you. We also explained to her that if you decided that you did not like someone that you would be unwilling to do anything that person asked you to do. It seems, though, that we are only parents. We have not been to school to learn how to teach special needs children, and just being with a special needs child 24/7, they felt did not qualify us to advise them on what techniques to use to teach you.

One day, she was trying to get you to look at her, and you wouldn't because you didn't like her, so she grabbed you by the chin and forcibly turned your face towards her. You *still* would not look at her. You looked everywhere but at her! I was pretty upset that she had manhandled you the way that she had, so I told her to never grab you by the face like she had again. I told her that you were very perceptive to tones of voice and facial expressions. I told her that you had proven time and time again to me that you understood everything that was being said. I told her that you were probably thinking that you were in trouble. I told her that all that she needed to do was to put her hand gently on the side of your face and *gently* turn your head towards her. I gained yet another enemy. But it was getting easier and easier for me to speak my mind without the restraint of caring whether or not the person being spoken to would like me or not following the exchange.

I finally had the opportunity to put her in her place when a news program aired on TV about a special school for autism in Los Angeles. The show followed the progress of the director's eight-year-old son who attended this school that followed a program developed by the mother of an autistic child in India. At the end of the program, when the little boy was asked how he knew so much, he replied, "All this time, when nobody thought that I was paying attention, I was actually listening." I had voiced almost those exact words with regard to you when you had first entered her classroom!

I found myself having to stand up to "professionals." Those "professionals" felt that since they had been to school for years, they had all of the answers. Albert Einstein once said that anyone who believes that they know everything is a fool. I strongly believe that.

I was constantly having to take a stand against building owners, schools, hospitals, corporations, and doctor's offices whom, because of you, I found were not being ADA-compliant. When they refused to right these particular wrongs, with the help of CEO's offices, school superintendents, and my elected officials, they were forced to do the right thing. It was because of you that things that made it harder for other disabled people to navigate the world were changed and their ability to navigate the world improved.

When you got really sick at the end, I kept telling the doctors about my family history and what I felt they should be checking for. They did check for it but used the wrong test. When I said that I really felt that I was right about what was going on with you, they repeated the same test ... eight times. I finally said to the doctor in front of doctors that he was training, "Do you know what the definition of insanity is? It is doing the same thing over and over and expecting different results." I then suggested a different test. They finally performed that test and found exactly what I had been telling them I thought was the problem all along.

When you finally got out of the hospital, you needed extensive therapies to try to get you back to the place that you were before the hospitalization. The thing is, though, that you have to find that therapist that truly believes in their patients and listens to the parents. Your speech therapist never gave up on you, and you made a great deal of progress with your ability to swallow. Your physical and occupational therapists, though, kept giving up on you, siting their belief that you had reached your maximum potential. I argued with them and told them that your maximum potential would be your being able to do all the things that you had been able to do before your hospitalization. They were quite offended that I had the audacity to question their "expertise."

When the first physical therapist gave up on you, I started doing exercises with you that just required common sense. We called the agency back when I felt that you should resume your physical therapy, after getting a prescription from your doctor for this. This particular physical therapist refused to even come out and evaluate you. I then called the CEO of the company and explained the unprofessionalism of this individual and they sent out a different physical therapist, one who believed in your ability to reach your maximum potential per my description of what your maximum potential was, which was what you had been able to do prior to being hospitalized.

There was one occupational therapist who refused to listen to me and obviously did not believe in you. She discontinued your therapies twice, saying that you had reached your maximum potential. I argued this point, saying that your maximum potential was you being able to have the full use of your body, just like you did before being hospitalized. I told her, as I had told the previous physical therapist, that it is just common sense that when someone plateaus, you just change gears and switch things up. She continued to argue with me, so I asked her if tomorrow she found herself in a hospital bed for five months, what she would expect her maximum potential to be, barring neurological damage, and she said that she would expect to be able to do everything that she could do at that time. I then asked her why it should be any different with you. She could not give me any kind of credible explanation and then proceeded to leave, her face revealing the huge amount of anger that she felt at me for contradicting her. I was then left to try to figure out how best to help you get back to the you that you had been. I succeeded in part but then called the agency back a few months later to reestablish services. We asked for a different person since we knew that this particular therapist had no faith in your recovery, but they still sent her back and we went through the same struggles with her. I could never give up on you, honey. I knew that you were frustrated with not being able to do the things that you had been able to do, so I kept pushing on. You were never a quitter and I could not bring myself to quit on you.

You Taught Me about Human Cruelty

You taught me how cruel people can be to those who are different from them. It is not that I didn't always know this, but it becomes so much clearer when this is personally experienced. I don't know why you felt that this was something that I had to become so personally versed in, but I will have to trust that you knew that this was something vital to my development as a "humane" being, something that I have found a large number of human beings are not.

You began this particular lesson with the medical community, specifically doctors. People are made to believe, primarily by doctors themselves, that doctors are superior to everybody else. We are told about the Hippocratic Oath and that their job is to first do no harm. The actions of some of your doctors led me to question to whom they felt they were doing no harm. Their actions made me draw parallels between the supposed meaning of the Hippocratic Oath and the definition of hypocrite.

Your pediatrician referred us to a neurologist at the children's hospital when you were three months old because she was concerned about your muscle tone and episodes of screaming, so we made the trek to investigate this. The day of the appointment, we made the hour-long trip to this doctor's office and filled out the necessary paperwork.

We were then led into an examination room to wait for the doctor. When he finally appeared, he had that classic "mad scientist" look. His hair was greasy and unkempt. He had on dark-rimmed glasses that were a style popular in the 1940s and 1950s. He had on a yellow sweater-vest with black and yellow diamond shapes across the front over a white shirt. And he had a pocket protector with a few pens sticking out in the shirt pocket.

He spent no more than three minutes examining you and then said to Daddy and me, "My advice is for you to get rid of him before you get attached. You are young. You can start over. He will never walk, talk, or show emotion."

I guess I was more shocked than Daddy because I was speechless, whereas Daddy backed this doctor up against the wall. I got you dressed, picked you up, and held you close to me. So many thoughts were swirling through my head. I kept thinking, *Wow, this is a case of throwing the Hippocratic Oath in the toilet.* You were the one who was his patient, not Daddy or me. How could he possibly think that your parents throwing you away would cause you no harm? I figured that he must have, when in medical school, missed all of his Bedside Manner classes, an area that he obviously needed to work on.

Years later, we met a mother of a little girl with chronic neurological problems and found out that this doctor was also this child's doctor. Listening to this little girl's mother tell the story of her encounter with this doctor, it became apparent to me that he treated all of his patients with chronic neurological problems with virtual disdain. I could only wonder why someone who is obviously unable to tolerate children with chronic neurological conditions would choose a profession where he would be forced to deal with children with chronic neurological conditions. I was forced to come to the conclusion that it was financially motivated. He obviously couldn't care less about these children, but since their conditions were chronic, he would have a steady flow of income for years to come, so he would deal with the obvious revulsion that he felt when encountering them.

I always hoped that I would be able to one day bring you back to see him and show him that you had made it over all of the hurdles that he said would stand in your way, but we never totally reached that point.

We were to have insult added to injury years later by the doctor that we took you to for treatment of autism. We had been taking you to see this doctor for a couple of years, personally shouldering the cost of the treatments because the insurance companies did not pay for these treatments, based on the opinion that they are considered experimental. As far as I am concerned, most medicine is experimental. Otherwise, there would only need to be one medicine for each ailment, or better yet, cures would be found to replace the Band-Aids currently offered by the pharmaceutical industry and the medical world. We had given this doctor tens of thousands of dollars over the course of your treatment.

I remember you and Daddy coming home from an appointment with him and Daddy telling me that he had just spent three thousand dollars. I felt my heart drop down into my feet. No matter how hard or long we worked, we just couldn't catch a break. I had been working when I got this news, and since I worked at home, I just turned back around in my chair and resumed working.

The last time Daddy took you to see this doctor, he explained to him that we still wanted to see him, but would need to cut back on the frequency of the appointments because we could no longer afford to see him as often. The doctor's response was, "Don't you love your child?"

It was a good thing that it was Daddy that this was said to. He is the political one and I am the one who is confrontational, a condition acquired since your teachings began. How dare he question our love for you? I wonder how many other parents he had said this to. I wonder how many parents left his office wondering if they did indeed love their child as much as they thought that they did. I wonder if they were thinking that surely if they did love their child, they would be able to find the money to continue treatment, leading them to the conclusion that they must not love their child as much as they had thought that they did. I wonder how many parents left his office feeling like failures.

When you were about nine, I had to take you to see an ENT doctor whom you had not seen before because your doctor had cut back his hours. This doctor was young, definitely not long out of medical school, and was obviously a "God complex" doctor. When we finally got led into our little room, I explained to him that you had had a hoarse voice for over a month, following a bad bout of pneumonia.

He snickered at me! And then he said, "Well, he hasn't said anything while I've been in here. How do you know he has a hoarse voice?" He then gave me this demeaning look and sneered at me. I swear that I wanted to rip that smug look right off of his face but settled for giving it right back to him. I said, "*Unlike* you or I, he can't tell me with words, but *like* you and I, if he has a hoarse voice, this will become evident when any sounds come out of his mouth." I could tell the doctor was ticked off. His face totally lost expression and I could see the anger in his eyes. I didn't care, though. He had taken a demeaning, sarcastic stance with me, and I had taken just about as much as I was going to take from people like him.

He was probably just too young and inexperienced to believe that a mother, someone who spends most of their child's waking hours with them, would possibly know their child better than someone who had been learning via books for the past ten years. He was probably one of those doctors who believes that everyone fits into neat little categories per his books and that theory is more applicable than experience.

We had always liked the original doctor in this practice, which is the only reason that we had stayed with this office but had not thought that the members of his staff were worth much. There was this one woman with greasy, wavy hair who had an obvious problem with disabled children. She always looked at you like you were a freak. I know now that I should have said something to the doctor, but we had liked the doctor so much that we had not wanted to cause any problems.

Daddy came home from taking you to see this doctor one time and told me of an incident that had occurred while there. He said that there had been this woman there with her two children. You had been sitting on his lap reading a book and had not been bothering anyone. Daddy said that this woman kept staring at you like you were an alien. He had finally tired of the staring and had asked her if he could help her with something. She had immediately taken offense, gone up to the greasy-haired woman who worked at the desk and, I assume, complained about you and Daddy. The employee immediately shot Daddy a dirty look. Daddy probably at that point should have asked if there was a problem. We should probably have gotten the doctor involved. You and Daddy had done nothing, and yet this woman had claimed to be a victim when the truth of the matter was you and Daddy were the true victims.

Whereas I had not expected to be mistreated by doctors, I was not real surprised when attacked while out in public, although I do have to admit to being shocked at the nature and presentation of the attacks.

We had to fly north for a wedding when you were one and a half years old. We had brought your car seat, which was FAA-approved, so that you would be safely seated on the plane and also so that we would have a car seat for you while we drove around while visiting. Your little legs stuck out straight because your thighs weren't long enough. I sat by the window, Daddy sat in the aisle seat, and you sat in the middle so that should you have a seizure, one of us could hold you and the other could get you hooked up to the oxygen.

Shortly after takeoff, a stewardess approached us and made a comment about your feet almost touching the seat in front of you. I didn't think anything about this because both Daddy's and my knees were "just about" touching the seat in front of us, as the airlines cram as many seats as possible on the planes. A steward approached us within minutes of the stewardess leaving.

He was all militant-looking with a buzz cut and sharp features. He looked at us, put his hand on his hip, and said very loudly, "I don't like this at all!" We asked him what it was that he didn't like, and he said, "Well, his feet are 'just about' touching the seat in front of him. What would happen if someone needed to get out in an emergency?" We pointed out that our knees were "just about" touching the seats in front of us as well as the fact that there were just the three of us in the row and our seats were not in an emergency exit row. He again said even louder, "I don't like this at all!" We then attempted to explain to him that we needed to have you between us so that we could get you breathing again should you have a seizure. He was so thick that he just couldn't seem to comprehend what we were saying.

This occurred at a time when airline passengers were having confrontations with the stewards/stewardesses, so I think that he was trying to lay the groundwork to present himself as a victim of uncooperative passengers in an attempt to get himself in the newspaper or on television. I have never been able to come up with a better explanation for his behavior since we were not inconveniencing or endangering anyone, and there was no way, come hell or high water, that if something had happened, we would have just crawled over you and left you on the plane.

When we tried to explain a third time, he said to us in a very sarcastic manner, "Well, with his medical conditions, maybe he shouldn't be flying." Daddy started to say something, but I advised him that it was time to halt the conversation, as this guy was a complete moron. We were forced to move you next to the window. The steward then proceeded to ignore us the remainder of the trip.

When we got off of the plane, a few of the other passengers came up to us and apologized for the behavior of the steward. They gave us their names and business cards, saying that they would testify for us should we decide to pursue any legal action against the airline. When we were flying north a few years later, as luck would have it, this same steward was on our flight. He again paid us no heed, but Daddy overheard him telling the other stewardesses that he had done nothing wrong on that previous flight that we had been on.

You never bothered anybody when we were out in public. You minded your own business. You did your own thing, and yet people of all ages still went out of their way to attack you. I remember one day when we were playing on the playground across the street from our house. A little boy came up to me and said, "He's weird!" I know that I didn't give a very mature response to this when I said, "Well, maybe he thinks that you are weird," but I was so sick of people's stupid and cruel remarks that the words had seemed to just leap uncontrolled from my mouth.

There was another incident that occurred when Daddy was in the park with you. You were playing with Daddy when you noticed that some children had entered the park. Upon seeing them, you started laughing and running towards them. These children's mothers saw you coming, rounded them up, and herded them away from you, all the while looking at you as if you had three heads. I wish that I had been there because I would have taken your hand and followed them until they left the playground, and if confronted, which I would have hoped to be, I would have asked these women how they would like it if their children were to be treated like freaks were something to happen to one of them that made them irrevocably different than they currently were.

Daddy said that afterwards, you looked at him with eyes reflecting not only confusion but also deep sadness. I had seen a similar look on your face when we had been playing and two little boys came racing onto the playground, laughing. I had watched your face light up when you saw these boys and had then seen happiness replaced by sadness as they paid you no attention.

One time, when you were six or seven years old, we had gone out to eat at one of your favorite restaurants. We had finished eating and were making our way out of the dining room. You had been extremely well-behaved, as you always were when we went out to eat, watching your DVD player while being fed your meal. You hadn't made a peep, except for occasionally laughing at the parts of your DVDs that you found amusing. I had, in the meantime, listened to other children screaming and crying and watched as parents chased their children after they had gotten down out of their chairs and run around the restaurant. You, being good as gold, just sat in our booth. Daddy took you when we got up to leave, so I took your oxygen tank and the leftovers.

I was kind of surprised that Daddy had let me take the oxygen tank because I had accidentally hit an old man on the head with it the last time that we had gone to this restaurant. I had been trying to maneuver between the tables, which had barely enough room for a person to get through, and had knocked something off a table. I had quickly turned around to see what had fallen. When I stood back up after picking up the condiment rack that had fallen, I noticed an old man shooting daggers at me with his eyes. I was at a loss at that time to figure out why he was giving me that look. It wasn't until we got out to the car that I figured out that I had side-swiped him with the oxygen tank.

But I digress. So Daddy took you and I led the way through the maze of tables. When we got in the car, Daddy asked me if I had heard what the people at one of the tables had said. When I told him that I had not, he told me that someone had said, "I don't know why they don't just leave him at home." I was livid, honey! I wanted to go back into the restaurant and confront those people, but Daddy was dead set against me doing that.

The people at the table, if my memory serves me well, were "cotton tops." I wish that I had been the one to hear them say that because I would have turned around and called them on the carpet for their unconscionable behavior right then and there. I would have challenged them to repeat what they had said and then reminded them that they were at that age when strokes occur. I would have asked them that if they suddenly found themselves challenged medically, they would like to be shut up in their house forever, never to return to the public eye because they might offend someone's sensibilities. I believe that Daddy knew there would have been a confrontation while inside had I heard them make the remark about you.

I was sick-to-death tired of the ignoramuses of the world from whose mouths spewed cruel, uninformed, and unempathetic drivel and who seemed to take such delight in kicking someone when they were already obviously down. I found myself disgusted with the human race ... and the insults just kept coming. There were a couple of incidents that occurred in the grocery store. The first happened when you were about three years old.

I had you sitting in the child's seat part of the cart as I pulled up to the checkout counter. The cashier, an older woman, was flirting with an older man who was standing in line at the next checkout stand. She was obviously distracted by this and was feeling inconvenienced at having to ring me out while she was trying to hook up with this man. She was having trouble scanning my groceries, so I jokingly said, "They must be free today!" She gave me a dirty look and said, "No." She tried again but continued to have trouble, so I said, "See, I told you, they're free today." You were sitting in the cart making your little singsong noise. She looked at you and said in a very derogatory tone, "What is that, a monkey?" Everything seemed to stop at that moment. I looked at her, then the bag boy, and then you. The bag boy said, "Well, that was mean!" I turned to you, hugged and kissed you, paid my bill, and left, thinking at that time that this was not a fight I wanted to get into at that time.

    I couldn't let it go, though. Every time I thought back to what she had said and how she had said it, I found myself getting more and more angry. When the anger turned to tears, I knew that I had to do something about it. I figured that if she had attacked us unprovoked, then she would not hesitate to attack someone else. I had been given the opportunity to explain to her that her behavior was unacceptable and prevent someone else from having to suffer the sort of attack that we had just endured. I called the store's corporate offices and explained what had just transpired, still so angry that I was unable to turn off the tears.

    I got a call back from the store where the incident occurred within five minutes of hanging up the phone. I again explained what had happened, still unable to fight back the tears. I went into the store the next day to identify the lady. I then proceeded to the office. The woman was pulled off the register and brought to the office. She denied everything, saying that she couldn't remember having said anything untoward. I told her that it was really sad that she was unable to remember having hurled such an egregious insult at an innocent child, so I had to assume that this was how she ordinarily treated her customers. She continued to deny the accusation. I went on to tell her about you and the things that you had to go through on a daily basis, both medically and socially. She sat there with a blank expression on her face (maybe an excellent example of the saying, "Lights on but nobody's home"). I would have liked for her to be fired so that other disabled customers would not have to endure mistreatment at her hands, but the store manager refused to do this.

    I had another confrontation in the same store years later while I was shopping during the Christmas season. I had you sitting in the cart and was talking to you, as I had always done. I was making a special cake for your one-on-one at school and, since I rarely made this cake, was having to scan the shelves for the ingredients. I had reached a shelf where I thought that I would find a particular ingredient that I needed.

I scanned the shelf, not finding was I was looking for, and then began to steer my cart away. It was then that I heard a female voice say, "Why don't you stop talking to the fucking retard and move your ass?" I was so shocked that I couldn't move for a few seconds!

Then when I had managed to pick my jaw up off of the floor, I turned around and looked in the direction from which the insult had been hurled. It was a woman, probably in her twenties, dressed in Daisy Duke shorts, which barely covered her derriere. The rest of us were dressed in long pants and coats, as it was one of the rare times when the temperature had dropped to near-freezing. I moved my cart to the opposite side of the aisle, parked it, glanced at my watch, and stood with my arms across my chest, waiting for her to turn around. I waited and waited and waited and waited and then looked at my watch again. Five minutes had passed! I know that I had not been standing in that spot for more than thirty seconds before she had felt it necessary to insult us.

I waited another minute longer, finally realizing that she was one of those people who are too much of a coward to insult someone to their face, being much braver when uttering obscenities behind a person's back. I turned to you and said very loudly to ensure that she would hear me, not caring who else did, "Joseph, do you think that I should tell her to *kiss my ass*?" I then looked back at her to see if she had the cojones to confront me. As expected, she did not! She just stood in the same spot, watching me out of the corner of her eye, waiting for me to leave.

I immediately felt ashamed that I had gotten down into the gutter with her, ashamed that I might have embarrassed you, so I apologized to you for my behavior. She took this opportunity, while I was talking to you, to rush by me but not before giving me a sideways, crinkle-nosed glance. I had to physically stop myself from again insulting her. I do apologize if I embarrassed you, but my patience was wearing real thin with regard to the unkind insults hurled our way, and I found myself, more often than not, switching into a confrontational mode with very little impetus.

When I told people about the confrontation and what I had said, they applauded me. They told me that those kind of people need to be put in their place, something not near enough people were willing to do. That made me feel a little better about my actions. I always ended up feeling that I should have handled a situation in a more dignified manner after I got down in the mud and rolled around with an aggressor.

I initially tried to give people the benefit of the doubt. When people would stare at you, which I had always been taught was rude, I would look them straight in the eye and say, "He is autistic and has a seizure disorder." I wanted to give them the opportunity to learn about you and your conditions, hoping to dispel their ignorance and fear. People were sometimes open to learning but, more often than not, just turned and walked away, hopefully feeling properly chastised. Either way, I hoped that the encounter had taught them something.

The incident with strangers which I found inspired the most shock in me again occurred at a grocery store. You had been presenting me with all the signs that you were going to have a major seizure. I decided to go to the store to pick up some things, hoping that I would beat the onset of the attack. I misjudged! I had you sitting in the shopping cart so that I could get through the store as quickly as possible. I had just paid for the groceries and had made my way out the door when you went into a seizure. I pushed the cart up against a stone pillar so that it wouldn't roll away with my groceries, lifted you out of the cart, and laid you on the ground so that I could work to get you breathing again. I was not paying attention to anything but you at that point.

I yanked down your pants, inserted the Diastat, and put the oxygen mask on you. I then did what I always did when you had a seizure—I kissed your face, told you how much I loved you, and begged you to come back to me. People coming out of the store were gathering around and watching. A male nurse came out of the store and stayed with us until it was over. I always hated being in the midst of people when you had a seizure. I was much better at handling these things in a private setting. I think that the fear that I saw in people's eyes when I saw them watching your body convulse amplified that fear that I was already feeling.

You could have knocked me over with a feather when I noticed that our groceries had been taken. While I had been kneeling on the ground not two feet from the shopping cart, frantically trying to get you breathing again, someone had taken the opportunity to walk off with my purchases! I am not sure that I had ever felt that much disgust in my life! My opinion of human beings took another nosedive.

There was another incident that occurred while I was pushing you along on your tricycle one day, trying to teach you how to ride. I noticed an older woman pushing two small children in a stroller. I heard one of the children say, "Why is she pushing him on the bike?" I then heard the woman say, "Because he is lazy." As I walked by her, I looked her in the eye and said, "He is autistic and has gross motor skill problems." She quickly averted her eyes, picking up her pace as she hurried away. I can only hope that she walked away feeling as ignorant as she had shown herself to be.

Another time, I had you in a cart at a grocery store when an older woman approached me and told me what a lazy boy you were! So once again, I had to explain that you were autistic and epileptic, with difficulty walking due to low muscle tone and seizures. She immediately apologized, but I couldn't help but think, *Why do people always feel that it is their right to offer their uninformed opinion with regard to anything. Why can't people just keep their mouths shut when confronted with a situation that they know absolutely nothing about? Why can they not wait to offer their opinion until they have learned the reasons behind someone else's actions, giving that person or those persons the benefit of the doubt with regard to their reasons for doing something?*

It is bad enough when a stranger is cruel, but when it is someone whom you have known for a long time, someone whom you think is your friend, someone whose cruelty is totally unexpected, someone that you love, the cruelty is even more painful.

There was this little boy that you had known since you were about three years old. You saw something in him the first time that you met and only grew to love him more as time went by. When the two of you were little and the differences not as pronounced, you would chase each other around the house in your Flintstone cars. But as you got older and the differences became more obvious, he didn't want to have much to do with you. When forced to come to the house with his mother, he would spend his time trying to stay away from you. You loved him so much, though, that you did not recognize this avoidance as repugnance. Whenever you saw him come through the door, your face would light up like a Christmas tree. You would get up from whatever you were doing to run to him and greet him in the only way that you knew how, thinking that he was your friend.

This particular time, you had gone up to him and were pushing and pulling him, which I know could be annoying, but it was what you did and anyone who had ever been around you had known that. He then moved away from you. You proceeded to chase him around the house. It was what you had always done, so you had no idea that the rules had changed. Yet even if the rules had changed, you could only do what you could do. You were unable to modify your behavior at the drop of a hat, while he was quite capable of doing this if he chose to. Change in behavior, for you, had always been something that needed to be gradually introduced until it was no longer change but familiar.

I was sitting at the table with his mother, talking, when I heard this little boy whom you had known most of your life, whom we had tricked ourselves into believing was truly your friend, say, "Get that thing away from me."

I immediately ran to you. The smile of delight that had been on your face upon seeing him had disappeared. In its place was a look of utter shock and incredible pain. Looking at you, I felt as if I, too, had been unexpectedly attacked. Your beautiful little face was a canvas of absolute sadness. I felt my heart breaking for you. You then, with bowed head, walked over to the couch and sat down, an air of total rejection surrounding you.

I foolishly made a decision to let this incident go at the time, thinking that maybe this boy was having an off day, and believing that it was best not to acknowledge the behavior. I was made to regret that decision a week later when he repeated this behavior. I have to assume that my silence had made him think that his actions were acceptable. Lesson learned.

I was then forced to confront his mother, who insisted that she had not heard what her son had said, although she had been sitting next to me at the table in both instances and I had heard it loud and clear. I told her that if her son could not treat you nicely when in our house, I could not allow him to come in any longer. I told her that our house is your refuge from the rest of the world, where people display no qualms about making those different from themselves feel useless and unworthy, and that I would not allow that kind of behavior entrance into your sanctuary.

She proceeded to handle this situation like she and her son were the victims and that I had made her feel like they were "bad people." It is amazing how the guilty can twist situations in their minds so that they can feel that it is they who have been victimized! I believe that this was the attack that was the most painful for you, but it was just one of many examples with regard to finding out how people in our lives truly saw us.

I remember Daddy coming home one day with a story about how a store manager had said, "Did you guys see that fucking retard?" after noticing a little handicapped boy in a wheelchair. He knew all of us. He hadn't seen Daddy so hadn't known that he was within hearing range. Daddy said that this man turned several shades of purple when he turned and saw him. I have to assume that he was embarrassed at having been caught uttering such a despicable, uncalled-for remark. Daddy said that this little boy had been doing nothing. He had been sitting in his wheelchair next to his mother at the end of the checkout lane, waiting for his father to cash out. His only crime was apparently being severely disabled.

I knew then that this was probably exactly what this man thought about you, honey, regardless of anything that he had said or how he acted when you were around. I wondered what would inspire anyone to say something like this.

I believe that when people do something or say something, that thing that is said or done provides some kind of benefit for them. I, for the life of me, though, could not even begin to imagine what benefit verbally attacking, albeit from a distance, a physically or mentally-challenged person could provide a person. I could not imagine how kicking someone who is obviously down could possibly lighten the kicker's load. Every time I saw this man after learning of this incident, I saw through the façade and knew that I would never again be able to take anything that he said with any grain of truth or integrity, adding to the general distrust that I had with regard to people and their motives.

There had been a lot of signs along the way that these people were not our friends, but I had refused to acknowledge those signs. I am not sure why. I suppose that I still sometimes just wanted to fit in, so I felt that the occasional mistreatment was acceptable.

I had a teacher in my senior year in high school who had told us that we would be lucky if we had one true friend in our lifetime. She said that most people were fair-weather friends and would only be there when it served their purposes to be there. When the situation no longer served their purposes, they would be gone like yesterday's garbage. I hadn't believed her at that time but over the years found that she was spot on. People use people. It is just the way that human beings are wired. I wish that I had allowed myself to believe her words at the time that she had spoken them. Had I, we would not have made decisions based on other people's welfare and not our own, which eventually proved to be detrimental to us. Another lesson learned.

The incident that probably came as the most of a surprise to me was one that occurred at church. A church was the one place that I thought you, we, would be safe from attacks. It is, after all, the house of God, and the people who enter its doors are supposed to be people of God, kind and compassionate … Christians, right?

We had gone to church to attend the Christmas Eve service. These services were always something to look forward to. This service was absolutely amazing and we looked forward to being a part of it every year. The music was heavenly (no pun intended). They always seemed to get someone from the regional philharmonic orchestra to perform a couple of pieces of music.

We had arrived late because Daddy had gotten out of work late. We had come in through the back of the church and were cutting through the narthex to go to the "living room," where they had installed closed-circuit TV so that parents of children with disabilities could observe the service and not disturb the rest of the parishioners.

You always loved church music, and as soon as you heard it, you started "singing." Then you noticed the people. You had just started saying, "Hey," and "Hi," so when you saw the people, you looked right at them and said, "Hi! Hi! Hi!" I saw them look at you with what I would describe as disgust. They looked at you like you had done something that was truly abominable and inappropriate. You correctly interpreted their looks. I watched as the smile disappeared from your face, you stopped talking, and your gaze dropped to the ground.

We then proceeded to the "special" room to watch the service. I started to weep as I sat there, and the harder I tried to stop, the more I tried to convince myself that their actions meant nothing to me, the harder the tears seemed to flow. This was supposed to be a joyous time, a time when people put their best foot forward, a time when people were giving and compassionate. I think that I was numbed by this encounter. You had, again, presented the world with the absolute sweetness that you were. You had offered up a smile brighter than the sun at high noon. You had allowed them to hear the music that was your voice. And you had been rejected by the human race once again.

I was left to again wonder why. I was again to question whether they had any idea of the hurt that they had inflicted on your beautiful soul. And I wondered if the church was truly God's house and he had been present, if he would find some way to give these people that had so offended you a personal lesson to bring the point home to them.

I loved our church and I loved our minister. There were times when we would not have made it through financially had our minister not offered to help us. I was, though, very disappointed when he refused to speak to the congregation about this incident, if only to remind them that if there is a God, we are *all* God's children, that we all deserve to be treated with love and respect.

You didn't speak again for a month and three days. Your teacher had approached us about this about a week after it happened, telling us that you had not been talking at all. They questioned whether something had happened. I have to believe that those people at the church had made you sincerely believe that you had done something unforgivably wrong and, being the good boy that you were, you didn't want to make that mistake again. Since having you, it has been completely obvious to me that people need to be periodically reminded to behave humanely towards their fellow human beings, most especially towards those people who are towing a heavier load.

I have found that people have this innate need to bemoan their situations, even when it is pretty apparent to others that they really have nothing to complain about. The complaints that people liked to share with us seemed to invariably be related to fatigue associated with the normal things that their children were doing. And whereas these people liked to vent with us with regard to their "problems," no one seemed to want to hear our complaints.

It might have been because when a mother would complain to me about how tired she was because she was running around after her toddler all day, which, by the way, was her only job, I would tell her that her child was doing exactly what she was supposed to be doing. I told her that she should get down on her knees every single night and thank God that her child was healthy and doing the things that she was supposed to be doing developmentally. I told her that she should be happy that she was not tired because she hadn't slept for a week because her child had been running a 104 degree temperature, or that she had to work twenty hours a day, or that she was running around taking her child to various doctors or therapists … or that she had to split her time between staying at the hospital with her child and staying up all night working. I wished that she could understand how exceptionally lucky she was.

It is not that I didn't understand that she was tired. I did. Children are little Eveready bunnies. They keep going and going and going. And we as adults don't have that same energy level that we had as children. I just could not empathize with her. I could only wish that *my* reason for being exhausted was simply because my child was doing all the normal things that children do. And since I didn't exhibit that "poor you" attitude that these people were obviously in search of, I got tossed out of the playgroup.

People like to present the façade that they are open-minded and accepting of differences. You helped me to see past that façade. This situation is not as dire as it used to be fifty years ago when the disabled were locked away in basements and back rooms, but the human race has a long way to go with regard to true acceptance of the disabled. People don't really want to be around someone with severe disabilities. Maybe it reminds them of the frailty of the human body, which is something that people just don't want to think about. Nobody wanted to listen to me talk about how scared I was each time I had to bring you back from a seizure, how I lived days on end with my heart in my throat as I nursed you through yet another dangerously high fever, how my very soul actually ached as I contemplated the very real possibility of losing you forever. Maybe knowing about all that you went through made their problems seem as insignificant as they really were. And they needed their problems to seem significant, so they set off to find someone with problems just as insignificant so that they could feel that their complaints were justified.

There were laws that existed in this country, a country that is supposed to have been founded on the principle of freedom for all, called the "ugly laws." They existed on paper in this country from the 1860s through the 1970s until a brave man named Richard Pimentel began his fight for the rights of the disabled. These laws banned people who were deemed "diseased, maimed, mutilated, or in any way deformed" from public places. The disabled could be forcibly removed from any place where their presence offended someone and arrested if they refused to leave. The last law was struck down in 1974 in Chicago. Based on our experiences, I believe that although they do not exist on paper, they still exist in the minds of people and will continue to exist until a way can be found to change the mentality behind mistreatment of the disabled.

I wish that all those people who had mistreated you would have attempted to get to know you, the "you" that Daddy and I know. I know that had they, they would have fallen in love with you, just like everyone who did take the time to know you. They would have seen a little boy brimming with life and love, with a strength of spirit rarely encountered in this world. They would have seen a little boy with courage second to none when facing chronic, debilitating medical conditions that would bring most people to their knees. They would see a world made up of people like themselves, people who would choose to treat you with unkindness because of those same medical conditions that made you different in a world filled with people who are afraid of "different." If they had taken the time, I think that they would have realized that they were in the presence of a hero of epic proportions, a person of innate greatness.

I wish that they would have taken the time to learn about you and us as a family. I wish that they would have, at least, entertained the idea that we loved you more than anything on the face of this earth, more than anything in all the universes that exist, imperfections and all. I have heard it said that God doesn't make mistakes. I wish they would have taken the time to understand the rage that we felt when people would unconscionably take the opportunity to attack you unprovoked. I wonder if they ever stopped to consider the pain that their unprovoked words and/or actions that person and/or the people who love them felt. I wonder if they will ever understand that they had just piled a whole lot more pain on a heart already bursting with pain.

When you were about seven, we got you into a neuorobiofeedback program where they would attach electrodes to your head and have you control games on a computer with your brain. The endgame was to lower the alpha, beta, and theta brain waves. You did this better and faster than doctors, professors, and others with high IQs were able to do. We were told that you were probably a genius with an IQ over 200, having a brilliant brain in a broken body. The thing is, people could not, or would not, see this. When they looked at you, I know that they were thinking, *The light is on, but nobody is home.* But the light was on and you were certainly home, as is the case with other people with disabilities. You understood everything that was said. You also correctly interpreted the looks in people's eyes when they looked at you and inflections in their voices when they spoke to or about you.

I found myself retreating more and more from the world, feeling a growing dislike for people in general. I found myself feeling condemnation for their pettiness and ignorance and cruelty. You, though, never failed to remind me that not all people are cruel or insensitive or selfish. I saw through you that good and kind people do still exist. I knew this in my heart, but the insults and cruelty seemed to leave a greater impression on my brain.

You Taught Me that There are Good and Kind People

I used to take you to healing services at a church near where we lived. Modern medicine had failed you and I was hoping that God might be willing to step in and present you with a miracle. I thought this unlikely, since I had never felt his presence in my life, but I prayed to him daily, begging him to heal you and, thus far, had received nothing. I was willing to go that extra mile and take you to "his" place in demonstration of my willingness to give him another chance to show us his mercy. Daddy came along once and one of your adopted grandmothers accompanied us a few times, but it was generally you and me.

We would arrive, be directed to the front of the line, and then bow before the priest, and I would silently plead with God for him to, this time, say yes to my request. We went to these services for a couple of years. Yeah, I know, I am thick-headed. It seems that I only have to be told no a few hundred times before I realize that the answer is not going to change to yes.

Anyway, after having been regulars at this service for quite a long time, your adopted grandmother came to the service with us. When we were before the priest, he told me that someone had left a gift for you, so I went with him and Grandma took you.

When I returned, you, Grandma, and an older couple were standing together. The man had tears streaming down his face. He looked at me and told me that he had been watching me take you before the priest for quite some time. He then cupped your face in his hands, pulled you to him, and said, "I love this little boy. I pray for him every day." I felt my heart swell with gratitude in response to his kindness. This is a reaction that you seemed to be adept at evoking in people who were willing to take the time to see with their hearts when responding to you rather than reacting from some other dark place in themselves where only hatred and prejudice reside.

One time, when we went to this service, as we waited to be signaled by the priest, you spotted this woman with long beautiful blond hair sitting in the front pew. You always loved hair. I am not sure why, but I imagine that you loved the feel of it. Anyway, you took notice of her hair, and as we got closer to her, you could not resist reaching out and yanking on her ponytail. You had acted so quickly that I had not had time to intervene. Her head jerked back, and she turned her head to see who had done this. I was mortified! I immediately began to apologize, explaining that you were autistic and had a fascination with hair. She handled this better than I had expected her to, just smiling and telling me that it was okay. You seemed to get away with things like this, whereas other people would have gotten a verbal, or possibly a physical, beating. I am not sure whether it was because of your beautiful face or that they recognized your differences and made allowances for them. Either way, I was thankful.

The people at Boston Market, where we were regulars, were always nice to you. Whenever we went into the local Boston Market, as soon as the people behind the counter saw you, they would call out, "Hi, Joseph!" One time, Daddy and you went there to pick up dinner. Daddy took his eyes off of you for a split second while you were standing in line, and you started "tickling" the hind end of the woman in front of you. Daddy said that he turned around immediately when he heard a woman exclaim, "Hey!" She first looked at Daddy, thinking that he had done this, and then at you when Daddy explained that you were not being fresh. He explained that she looked like his mommy and that you were just "tickling" her. You then went on to push the limits of personal interaction. You reached up to be picked up by her and lost your balance. Your hands landed on her breasts. I know that this was not intentional, it just happened that that was the part of her body that your hands made contact with as you attempted to break your fall. She thankfully handled this very well, simply saying, "And I thought that you were just an ass man." I was always thankful when people chose to react with humor instead of cruelty with relation to your innocent actions. You never meant anything bad; you just saw people as being a means to an end, there to provide for you should the need arise!

Another time, we had gone out for our daily after-dinner drive. We decided to take a walk inside the local CVS store. You had always liked to push the cart when in the store, and this provided an opportunity for you to exercise your legs. We were walking down an aisle when a woman came running up to us. She said, "I was pulling out of the parking lot and saw you drive in, so I turned around and came back." I just looked at her and smiled, wondering who she was and what she wanted. She said, "I met you two in Blockbuster, and we talked about your son and his conditions. I kept looking for you after that but never saw you again." I smiled and apologized for not recognizing her, explaining that I always talk about you and your conditions when given the opportunity in hopes that people will be willing to learn about autism and epilepsy but that I am terrible at remembering people." She smiled, then looked at you, and asked me if she could hug you. I told her that she could. She then looked at me and said, "I love this kid. I include him in my prayers every day." It seemed that these incidents always seemed to occur when my opinion of the human race was at its lowest.

Yet another time, we were in Blockbuster when a woman who had just exited the store looked back, saw you standing near the window, and came back into the store. She approached me and asked if she could hug you. She then turned to me and said, "Don't you ever give up on him."

There was another time in a grocery store when I noticed a man staring at us. I looked away, choosing to ignore him, thinking that he was just another rude "human," not caring how much discomfort he caused the object of his curiosity. I had gotten to the point where I generally did not look people in the eye in an effort to avoid giving people the opportunity to ignite any rage or disgust in me. I found that I either looked at the floor or directly at what I was searching for. He was still watching us when we walked by him, so I smiled and said, "Hi," at which point a conversation was initiated.

He explained to me that he had been watching us but had been unsure of whether or not he should approach us. He asked what was wrong with you, so I told him that you were epileptic and autistic.

This man had the most beautiful blue eyes! They glistened and were the color of the sky. He was being very kind, so I assumed that someone close to him was disabled. Experience had taught me that when someone was as compassionate as this man appeared to be, they had personally experienced the suffering of a loved one. When I asked him about this, he told me that his son had severe cerebral palsy.

As we spoke, I noticed tears beginning to spill from his eyes. This surprised me, but I figured that watching you, he was being reminded of his own pain. He then asked if he could hug me, and while he had his arms around me, he said, "I love you." I was taken aback a little bit by this at first, but as I looked into his eyes, I recognized the pain and sorrow residing there and knew that he understood what we were going through. I saw in him a rare kindred soul.

One day, Daddy, you, and I were out for a drive and came upon a carnival by the side of the road. We had pulled onto the carnival grounds simply to see if you liked or were afraid of the Ferris wheel. We were betting on the fact that you would like it because you always loved the wind in your face. We were right! You thought that you were pretty hot stuff, being way up high above everyone else. What we didn't expect, because we had come to expect mistreatment from others, was the kindness that the people working at this carnival showed us. When it got time to get off, the ride operator asked us if we would like to go again … for free … so we did!

Most of the ride operators at the carnival treated us with this same level of kindness, offering you free rides. The man operating the roller coaster presented us with a picture of you taken while on the ride. It was so funny! Your face reflected equal portions of terror and pleasure. When we passed by games that offered stuffed animals as prizes, they offered to give you the stuffed animal of your choice for free. We thanked them but declined, as you had never been particularly fond of those types of things. It was the thought that counted, though.

Daddy had taken you on most of the rides and then decided that it was my turn. The ride went backward and forward. Daddy and I thought that you would like this ride because it went fast and you always loved the feel of the wind on your face. You liked going forward on this ride but were not so keen on going backward. You went into a seizure near the end of the ride. The man operating this ride noticed that you were having a problem, and the second that the ride stopped, he was at the top of the ramp and at your side. He lifted you out of the car, as if you weighed nothing, and carried you to safety. Looking at this man, I would not have thought that he was strong enough to lift you with such ease, but he did! I was amazed at the goodness in his heart!

I'm not sure why we were the recipients of so much kindness on this day at this place, but I have to assume that it had something to do with the fact that society tends to look down on carnival people. The general population tends to view them as lesser beings maybe because they are transient. I believe that they saw kindred souls in you, Daddy, and me, people who judged others by the quality of their character with eyes whose judgment was not clouded by discrimination. What I witnessed that day was proof positive that these were people who possessed in their very souls the qualities that exemplify the best of what it is to be a human being. They showed kindness and compassion. They gave of themselves. They gave from their hearts. And that is the best that we as human beings can give.

One of the greatest gifts of kindness that we received was offered up by one of your adopted grandmothers. She gave us the money to take you to Lourdes for a healing, as she herself had been cured of end-stage colon cancer thirty years earlier. Daddy and I turned her offer down at first but then felt that we should not let pride get in the way of the possibility of a brighter future for you. We accepted her gift and flew off to France a couple of months later.

It was an amazing trip and again reminded me of the goodness to be found in the human race. We spent our first night in Paris and took a train to the south of France, to Lourdes, the next afternoon.

The people on the train seemed to be drawn to you, wanting to know all about you. You enjoyed all the attention given you. You, being the consummate traveler, loved the train ride. You sat quietly by the window, drinking in the sights passing by. We had quite a bit of luggage with us, and when we arrived in Lourdes, without our even having to ask, people we had been speaking with on the trip down picked up your luggage and carried it off the train for us! This was one of many kindnesses extended to us while in Lourdes as well as Paris.

Our main reason for going to Lourdes was to bathe in its "healing waters." You went with me, as you were a child, and Daddy went to the men's baths. We all had to strip down, then wrap a sheet around us, and wait our turn. Thank God the room was warm! When it was our turn, we shed our sheets, which were immediately immersed in the water, wrung out, and then wrapped around us. We then commenced to descend the stairs into the bath.

When your feet hit the water on the first step, you gasped because the water was so cold and lifted one leg up at the knee, pointing your toes like a ballerina. I had to force you to continue into the bath, with you gasping each time the water climbed higher up your body. We walked to the front of the bath and back. We were immediately wrapped in towels and then got dressed. We repeated the ritual the next day, with you having the same reaction. We should have gone a third time, but I felt selfish in wanting to do this, as there were hundreds of people waiting to have their turn in the baths

While in Lourdes, we decided to join the nightly candlelight procession on the grounds of the Church. We didn't think to consider that we should have a candle for this until we got there and saw that everyone else had a candle. It was too late to purchase one, though, because all of the shops were closed, but I decided that we were going to join the procession, anyway.

Within seconds of joining the procession, a man came up to us and gave us his candle. I guess he felt that we needed it more than he did. It started to drizzle not far into the walk. We had dressed you in a warm coat with a hood, but we had not thought to cover your legs. I immediately took off my jacket and put it over your legs. A woman walking near us must have seen me do this, as she came over and put her umbrella over you, leaving herself exposed to the rain. I felt like weeping at this unexpected kindness. When we left to go back to our hotel room, I was again reminded of how kind people can be when a man, seeing me pushing you in the wheelchair, offered to give us his umbrella. He didn't know us from Adam and yet had felt concern for a stranger's well-being.

We experienced this level of treatment everywhere we went in France. When Daddy had to ask people for directions in order to get something for you, those people walked a few blocks out of their way to personally take him where he needed to go and then brought him back to where they had first seen him. We were in a supermarket one day when you threw a hissy fit and bit Daddy. This caused a loose tooth to come out and your mouth to bleed. A man approached us within seconds with a wet paper towel to wash the blood away. It's funny to think that everyone had told us to fear the French, and yet the French, total strangers, had shown us a level of kindness unfamiliar to us back home.

When you were five, I wrote a letter to celebrities and heads of state telling them about you and asking them to write a letter of encouragement to you. We received quite a few letters in response, each of which I read to you. These people took time out of their busy days to give words of comfort to you, a stranger to them. I hope that receiving these letters made you feel proud and worthy, although sadly the best I will probably ever be able to do is surmise that they did.

One of the people who we had written a letter to and gotten a response from was Prince Albert of Monaco. When we had found out that we were going to France, Daddy had e-mailed him to tell him that we would be in Europe and would like the opportunity to personally thank him for his kindness in taking the time to pen a letter to you. Daddy was pleasantly surprised when he received a response from his staff asking what day would be best for us to meet with Prince Albert!

The morning that we arrived in Monaco, we were met by a man named Jean Marc, who had been assigned to be our escort while there. We started the day with a meeting with Prince Albert. He wasn't what I had expected him to be, considering his station in life.

He was very down to earth and kind. He spent about twenty minutes with us and presented you with some gifts.

We were then asked if we would like to see the changing of the guard. Jean Marc led us to the entrance of the palace where we joined hundreds of people waiting, cameras in hand, to witness the changing of the guard. We then watched as velvet ropes were put up, splitting the crowd in half, forming a path before us to the front of the palace. The head guard then marched towards us and escorted us to the front of the crowd. As we followed the guard, Daddy said that he had heard people asking who we were. He said that people had been taking pictures of us, as if we were people of importance! If they had only known!

Jean Marc then took us to one of Prince Albert's restaurants, and because you were on a special diet at the time, his chef prepared you a special meal. You just about inhaled it! This was the first time that you had really eaten with any gusto since we had arrived in Europe. While Daddy, Jean Marc, and I talked, I noticed you watching Jean Marc out of the corner of your eye. He didn't notice you doing this, but knowing you, I knew that you were sizing him up.

When we got up to leave the restaurant, as Jean Marc approached you, you took his hand and walked off with him. You had decided that he was a good egg. This, I am also sure, he did not realize was something monumental, as you rarely reached out to people. I had learned over the years that you were an excellent judge of character, having shown me time and time again that your like or dislike of someone should be used as a gauge to assess people. I only knew you to be wrong one time. You chose Jean Marc and stayed by his side whenever he was near.

Jean Marc was only the second person that you had ever left my side for, and whereas I had felt a bit hurt the first time you did this, this time I knew that you were not choosing him over me but that you had just found a humane being that you felt a connection with. He spent the rest of the day with us, informing us that we were his "job" for the time that we were in Monaco.

When we got back to our hotel, you had one of your bad grand mal seizures. You had started getting sick in Paris because it had been bitter cold, which is something you weren't used to. I, therefore, stayed at the hotel with you while Jean Marc took Daddy to Monte Carlo. He told me that when he arrived there, after he had told them who he was, they had said, "Hello, we have been expecting you." He was treated like royalty! We were *all* treated like royalty wherever we went in Monaco.

When Daddy got back from his unsuccessful experience gambling in Monte Carlo, we tried to get dinner sent up to the room because you were in a postictal phase, and we wouldn't have been able to rouse you for hours. We were told that the patrons of the hotel were not allowed to eat in the rooms. When the manager of the hotel got wind of this, he called the room to find out what had transpired, and when we told him that we would have to go down to the restaurant in shifts because you had had a bad seizure, he apologized to us over and over again. He then advised us that, of course, they would bring our meal to our room. I have to assume that he then advised Prince Albert of your condition because we received a call from the palace shortly afterward asking if you needed to be seen by his father's personal neurologist!

I am not sure whether or not Prince Albert will ever be able to fully realize what he did for us, aside from the obvious, with these simple acts of kindness. Here was a man who knew that we could not possibly give him anything in exchange for his kindness, and yet he had chosen to treat us as if we were important. His treatment of us was food for our battered souls, souls that had been under seemingly constant attack by man's inhumanity to man. There is no way that we will ever be able to properly thank him for treating us as if we, too, were deserving of the good things that life has to offer.

You Taught Me How Sweet Little Boys Can Be

I had always wanted to have a girl before you came along, but having had you, I would have gladly had a houseful of little boys had that been my destiny.

When you were little, you loved doing all the things other children find joy in doing. You used to zoom around the house in your Flintstone car, maneuvering around corners and turning at exactly the right time to slide through the bathroom door. You loved being in the bathroom for some reason, and when you were out of my sight, I knew I would find you lying on the floor in the bathroom reading a book. I figured this had to have some connection to males and their fascination with bathrooms.

You loved crinkling up your nose and making a "monster" face. You looked so cute when you did this! You loved going to the beach, enthralled by the crashing of the waves on the shore, and splashing in the water—that is, until you got slapped in the face by a breaking wave while you were laughing. You didn't like the ocean after that, preferring to kick around in the pool in your child's float and then, when you got too big for the floats, pull yourself around the edge of the pool.

You so loved going to the pool, and one day, your one-on-one called to say that he was right around the corner and would be there in a few minutes to take you swimming. I immediately got you dressed in your swimsuit and gathered everything that you would need. I then put your video on, but you stood waiting by the door, and I went back to work. I lost track of time and noticed that forty-five minutes had gone by and that you had stood by the door the entire time waiting for him to appear. When he finally did, I had a word with him and told him that I would never let him do that to you again.

The only other time that you waited by the door was when you saw Daddy and me getting dressed to go out, and since we had never gone out without you, you thought that we were all going someplace together. You were standing at the door when we approached, and we had to explain to you that we were going out and leaving you with a woman who had watched you when you were home from school and I had to work. A look of sadness came over your sweet face. You had a good time with this woman, but we felt so guilty about leaving you to go out on a "date night" that we never went out without you again. We were the Three Musketeers and could never do this to you again because you loved being together as a family.

You loved your walker and the freedom that it gave you to move around the house on your own. I remember you running around the house in your walker when you were a baby, sometimes going up to the screen door and pushing your face against the screen. Your cuteness never seemed to end! You also loved being around people, always trying to win them over with your sweet personality.

You loved your toys and would lie on the floor for hours at a time, pushing your favorite buttons on each toy. You had two pull-down music toys in your crib, and you would constantly pull them down when they stopped until you finally fell asleep. You especially loved your books, and when I was not reading them to you myself, you would lie contentedly on the floor, flipping through the pages of your various Dr. Seuss books. You also loved your videos, most of which were original Dr. Seuss, but the video that you liked best, the one that got you through many illnesses, was *Sebastian's Caribbean Adventure*. I would have to play it over and over all day when you were sick because it seemed to be the only video that you wanted to watch when you weren't feeling well. When you refused to get up from your nap, all I had to do was to put this video on and you immediately woke up and rushed to the TV to watch it!

You loved to go to the park to swing in the special needs swings and slide down the slide that was made with roller bars. You loved walking, running, and chasing me. I know you felt the loss of that particular freedom when you began having drop seizures, and we had to get you a wheelchair so that you would not fall and hurt yourself. You could still stand and walk, just not by yourself anymore.

Yours was an innately sweet soul aided by the fact that Daddy and I always smothered you with love from the get-go. You found joy in most everything, and when you laughed, your laugh came from your very toes! Your laugh was honest and contagious! It was hard for anyone to not laugh with you once you got going. You had that "pee your pants" kind of laugh.

I can't tell you how many times that when I went to pick you up from school, people that worked there would come up to me and tell me that you had started laughing and that they had been unable to stop laughing themselves. I guess it was like Barb at Easter Seals said, that people wanted to be around you because you got a kick out of everything. Love emanated from you. Whenever you saw me, Daddy, Grandma, or Grandpa, a smile would light up your face and you would extend your chubby little arms, requesting to be picked up and loved. There seemed to be, for you, joy in the simple act of being alive and loved. You always seemed to be able to find a reason to smile, even under circumstances that would have broken the average human being.

When you were a baby, I would rest my forehead against yours and look into your eyes while I gave you your bottle. I suppose that by doing this, I was teaching you that this was the way that this was done. Whenever I didn't do this, should I be talking to someone else, or not giving you my full attention while feeding you, you would try to catch my gaze, sometimes putting your hand to the side of my face and turning it towards you. Once eye contact was made, you would lift your head and move your forehead towards mine, showing me how it was properly done.

When you were just shy of three years of age, a special needs teacher named Katherine came to the house to work with you. She asked what you liked and I told her books. She laid down on the floor with you and started reading. When it came time to turn the page, she looked at you and said, "Turn the page." and you did. I had never said those words to you, but you understood exactly what she was asking you to do and continued to do it from that day on. You were so proud of yourself! You, after that, when lying on the floor reading, knew that you could read through any of your books all by yourself, with no help from anyone.

There was a period of time, after you had had secretin therapy, that you developed a fear of the dark. You had never had this fear. Bedtime had been relatively uneventful. When bedtime came, I would lay you in bed, cover you up, and turn out the light. However, after the secretin therapy, you would get up after I left the room. I would hear you "whining," and when I got to you, you would be standing up in your crib, looking at the animals on your wallpaper with a wide-eyed look of terror in your eyes. I stopped putting you in bed before you were asleep after witnessing this a couple of times. I began to hold you in my arms and rock you to sleep before putting you in bed. I loved this time, holding you in my arms, even though I knew that it would push my bedtime further into the wee hours of the morning. Those times when you just didn't want to go to sleep, we would get into my bed and I would pretend that I had fallen asleep. I would start to snore, softly at first, gradually getting louder, and occasionally snorting loudly. This would startle you and you would then start laughing when I did this. You always seemed to believe that everything that Daddy and I did was for your pleasure.

One night, Daddy came home late from work. You and I were deep in sleep. Your bed was right next to ours because we wanted to be able to get to you quickly should you have a seizure. Daddy said that he got into bed but didn't stay long. He said that I started snoring, and every time I snorted, you would start giggling. He tried, to no avail, to get me to stop snoring, pushing me onto my side. I continued to snore and snort and you continued to giggle. He gave up after about twenty minutes and went to sleep in the other bedroom.

You always had this James Dean thing going on. You saw yourself as being "bad" and were damn proud of it. I always played along with you on this because it always seemed to bring you such joy to think that you were truly wicked. I let you think that you were good at it, but you were really not quite the pro that you thought you were. You usually gave yourself away, giggling uncontrollably, just anticipating my reaction to your antics. I let you have your illusion, not letting on that I knew that you were about to try to put one over on me. You tried so hard to be coy and sneaky that I had to let you believe that you had succeeded.

Whenever you did most anything, I either pretended that you were being horribly evil or the most brilliant little boy ever to exist. This sometimes worked and it sometimes backfired. Either way, I had your attention and you were inspired to repeat your actions.

When you were a baby, I introduced you to the "tickle monster." I would shape my hand into a claw and start moving my fingers as my hand approached you, all the while saying, "Here comes the tickle monster!" You would start kicking your fat little legs and giggling uncontrollably. You quickly became adept at making your own tickle monster, but instead of coming after me or Daddy, you would go after yourself, laughing as you "scared yourself."

You then moved on to tickling other people. When you would tickle me, I would laugh harder and harder, and you would tickle harder and harder, all the while smiling from ear to ear. I loved having this interaction with you because I think that it made you smile from your heart and filled your very soul with gladness and a surety that you were loved to the fullest extent possible for one person to love another. That did not always work when you did it to unsuspecting people, but when they turned and saw your beautiful face and smile, they chuckled too!

In one of your favorite books, *Mr. Brown Can Moo, Can You?*, one of the sounds that Mr. Brown can make is "knocking." I always pretended that this was bad or scary, so that was what you came to associate this with. You would "knock" when you were angry. You did this when we were in Lourdes. You were trying to sleep and the group on our floor was making a lot of noise partying. This woke you, so you pounded on the wall to let them know that they were disturbing your beauty sleep. The same thing happened on the overnight train back to Paris from Monaco. Someone was making more noise than you felt necessary, so you again pounded on the wall to get them to quiet down!

When we were having new carpet installed in the hallway and upstairs bedrooms, the installers were making a lot of noise pounding. You, knowing the "knocking" was bad, kept giggling every time you heard a hammer come down. You probably thought that they were going to get into trouble for this activity and were laughing because you were glad that it was not you that was going to be in the hot seat.

You were always thankful, although I am not sure why since you rarely got in trouble for anything, when it was someone other than you that was getting in trouble. I think that this all started with *The Cat in the Hat*. I would always take on an angry voice when the Cat was doing something that he was going to get in trouble for with the mother. The mother, of course, always seems to be the punisher. Every time we came to a part where the Cat was getting himself into hot water, you would start giggling.

You demonstrated your joy in seeing someone else in trouble a number of times, but two occasions stick out the most in my mind. Daddy and you had gone to the ale house one night to pick up dinner. I think that you were about five at the time. Daddy had gotten you out of the car and was heading into the restaurant when he heard a commotion. He turned and saw a group of people standing around a woman basically beating a little boy. The little boy was about three. She was spanking him so hard on the butt that his little legs were going out from under him. The boy, of course, was screaming and crying. When you heard the boy crying, you started laughing. Daddy knew that you were not laughing because the boy was hurt, but because you thought that someone was in trouble. An elderly couple heard you laughing and told you that it was not very nice to be laughing in this situation. So as it seemed, we always ended up doing what we usually did when your behavior was in question—Daddy had to explain about you and the things that you did.

Another time that you laughed at the expense of someone else didn't end up working all that much in your favor. It was your first time at the dentist. When we arrived at the dentist's office, we were led to a small waiting room. It wasn't long before we heard a little girl screaming bloody murder. While other children would have been scared by this, you reacted differently. As soon as you heard the screaming start, you started running around the room laughing hysterically. Every time she screamed, you just laughed harder. It was all fun and games, hilariously funny, until it was your turn to go under that proverbial knife. It was then your turn to scream like a girl!

You were successful in some areas in your quest to be bad and test your parents' patience. One night, when you were about two, I had put you in bed and then gone back downstairs to work. I hadn't had my butt in my chair for more than a few seconds when I heard you pounding on the wall. I got up, pounded my way up the stairs, and turned the hall light on as I rounded the corner to your room. You were standing up in your crib. You just looked at me, as if to say, "What's up?" I went to you, laid you down, and told you to go to sleep. I then left your room, turning off the light on my way out, and went downstairs to finish up my work.

Again I hadn't been sitting for more than a few seconds when I heard you banging on the wall. I got up, pounded my way up the stairs, and turned on the hall light as I rounded the corner to your room. You were again standing up in your crib, a look of total innocence on your face. I again laid you down and instructed you in a sterner voice to go to sleep. I then left your room, turning off the light on my way out, and went downstairs to finish my work.

You still were not ready to go to sleep. I had a ton of work left to do before I could lay my head down on my pillow and I really needed for you to go to sleep. And you went for a third round. I have to admit that I was not happy at that point because all the interruptions were pushing my bedtime closer and closer to one in the morning. So … I got up again, pounded my way up the stairs, and turned on the light as I rounded the corner to your room. This time, though, as I reached the doorway of your bedroom, I watched as you threw yourself down on the mattress. You again looked up at me with that "Hey, Mom, what's up?" look on your face. The scenario did not prove to be in your favor. Your limbs were bent every which way, proof that you had quickly thrown yourself down on the mattress as you heard me approaching.

You always thought that you were the king of sneakiness! An example of this would be one night when I put you in bed and then went downstairs to watch a movie with one of your adopted grandmothers. I had hooked you up to your pulse oximeter, as we did every night. This device served as your Achilles heel with regard to making sure you got caught when you were trying to do your best sneaky maneuvers.

    I was sitting in the chair watching a movie with Grandma when my peripheral vision picked up something moving upstairs. When I looked closer, I saw a head full of curls advancing along the hallway floor. So I said, "Hey, are you out of bed?" You immediately stopped, and I saw the curls retreating back into the bedroom. I ran up the stairs and caught you combat crawling backwards in an attempt to get back into bed before I got to you! There were many times that you were successful at getting back into bed when the pulse oximeter alarm went off. I know that you thought that you were successful at covering your tracks after the alarm reported that you were on the move, but you usually got the cord to the machine caught on something on your way back into the bed and your leg would be stuck in a strange position.

    I have to admit to having enjoyed your attempts at being the bad boy. The sparkle that this would bring to your eyes was worth it. But possibly to your dismay, you were the sweetest human being I ever encountered, even considering your Dr. Jekyll/Mr. Hyde moments. You loved completely and hated to disappoint those people that you loved the most, especially me. When we fought, you always recovered much more quickly than I did. You never seemed to understand that I needed time after an attack to pull myself together. I had wounds to lick and a psyche to adjust. Even though you could not understand why I was still upset, you could tell that I was. That was another innate skill that you seemed to possess ... the ability to read people. You didn't like people to be upset, so you pulled out your "cute" arsenal to win back the affection that you feared you might have lost. I sometimes had to let you swim in that fear so that you would realize that what you had done was unacceptable and made me, if only for a short time, not like you. And I would tell you this when you tried to approach me. When I would gently push you away and tell you that "I don't like you very much right now," you would get a sad look on your face and sit down a short distance from me, all the while glancing over at me, waiting for me to give you a sign that the fight was officially over and that I loved you once again.

I knew that you were feeling remorse at having hurt me, but I sometimes needed to put distance between us. I remember one time that you had been particularly aggressive with me, so I went out into the kitchen. You followed me but did not approach me. You sat down at the table with *There's a Wocket in My Pocket*. I had always pretended that I was scared by the "vug under the rug," so to try to get me past my anger, you held the book up and started shaking it, pretending that you, too, were scared. I have to admit to that being one of the few times that you were able to "cute" me out of my anger! This particular book was one of your favorites, and at the end, you would always kiss the "zillow on the pillow" good night.

You had this therapist that you particularly loved, Paula, P.T. She loved you too! During one session at the house, she was trying to get you to go up and down the stairs. You had no problem climbing up the stairs but weren't real keen on coming back down the stairs on your own. Paula didn't let you get away with anything and refused to let you dictate the rules to her. I was, as always, sitting at my desk typing when I heard you start complaining and crying. I immediately got up and ran to the stairs, where I was promptly instructed by Paula to leave the two of you alone. You fought with her for twenty minutes, crying all the while, until you had her crying too. She wouldn't give up, though, and you finally came walking down the stairs. Both of your faces were tearstained and your eyes were swollen. The session time was up following this, so Paula left. You were upset the rest of that night as well as the next day, and the next time that she came to the house for your therapy, you approached her hesitantly, unsure of whether or not she was angry with you. Your face lit up when you realized that she wasn't mad, and from that day on, you always did whatever she asked you to do, afraid that she would not forgive you again.

Your love for those in your life was rock-solid, and I think that you felt the need to protect those people. I am certain that you assigned yourself as my knight in shining armor, viewing me as your personal damsel in distress. You took such pride and joy in this and the satisfaction that you experienced with regard to this was written all over your face.

We had a family portrait taken at our church when you were about three. We hung it proudly on the wall. I picked you up after we had hung the picture up and said, "Mommy, Daddy, Joseph." Every time we walked by that picture, you would put your little arms up, telling me to pick you up, and you would look at the picture and smile. I would always repeat those same words, "Mommy, Daddy, Joseph," and you would smile and put your little arms around my neck and give me a big hug. I wonder if you knew that this simple act made me smile with my heart. I hope you did.

We had laid mats on the floor so that if you had a seizure, you would have something soft to land on, and we would read your books, all of which you had memorized. I always acted them out to make them as interesting as possible. You would turn from looking at the book and look at me with a smile on your face, your eyes full of love, and then kiss my cheek and place your head against my shoulder. I would then put my head against yours, basking in the sweetness that was representative of the person that you were.

One time, right before we went to Brazil, Daddy and I were wrestling on the floor. You were lying on the floor a few feet away, reading. I called out to you to help me. When you heard my call for help, you looked our way and assessed the situation, thinking that Daddy was hurting me. You got up from the floor, walked over to us, threw yourself on top of Daddy, and bit him! You showed him once again that I belonged to you and only you and that you were willing to fight for your possession.

I found that I could use this "knight in shining armor" mentality to my benefit. Since you saw yourself as this strong alpha male providing protection and assistance to a needy ward, I would pretend to be frantic or scared, in need of your aid, so that you would come to me. You always answered my call. You would pop up from wherever you were and come running to me, giggling harder and harder the closer you got to me. You would then throw yourself into my waiting arms. Mission accomplished! "Saving me" always seemed to bring you such happiness and satisfaction that I gladly allowed you to think that you were my savior. And you probably really were!

You took great pride in helping me. I made a habit of making you think that I was very inept, although this was probably not far off the mark, as a way of tricking you into doing things for yourself. I would make grunting noises and start mumbling, complaining about how hard something was to do or how I was just incapable of doing something, and you would rush to my aid, "assisting" me with whatever task I appeared unable to accomplish. A look of such total satisfaction would wash over your face after you had "helped" me, so there is no doubt in my mind that the methods that I employed in feigning ineptitude truly worked their magic on you.

Maybe all that time I had been misreading your joy in helping me. Maybe you were really thinking how inept I was and wondering how I ever managed to get things done before you came along. I suppose that is another thing that I will never know for sure, as you lacked the ability to speak, and I could only make assumptions based on observations. Maybe you viewed me as being needy, and maybe I am, but know that I tried very hard to balance my need to see you experience joy with your need to grow as an individual.

Honey, I never wanted you to know that I had actually been in an almost constant state of panic since the day that you were born. I probably did not do as good a job as I should have at hiding this fact. I am not sure that this mattered, since you showed me time and time again how adept you were at reading in people those things that they didn't want the world to see.

You Taught Me to Never Give Up and Led Me on a Spiritual Journey

You were so sick all of the time, my love. We just couldn't seem to keep you well for any period of time. You were in the hospital pretty much one week out of every month, and it seemed that the other three weeks your little body was gearing up for its next hospital stay. It was exhausting! I was working all the time, trying to keep up with the bills and also provide you with any therapies and therapeutic products that we thought might help you. When you were sick at home or in the hospital, I had to find a way to get all of my work done so that we wouldn't lose my income, as we would have sunk much faster had I not been working. No matter how hard we worked, though, it seemed that we were just treading water, with the threat of drowning ever imminent. I was, in all actuality, operating on automatic most of the time, with little time to think of anything more than getting through each day.

Those rare times when a lull in activity would occur, I found myself feeling hopeless and thinking how futile our attempts were proving to be. It was at exactly those times that something traumatic would happen with you. You would be burning up with a fever, go into a seizure that would seem to last an eternity, or develop pneumonia. I would go into my emergency room physician mode, and when I had gotten you through yet another death-defying act, I would look into your beautiful eyes and see a soul that didn't know the meaning of the word defeat. I would see a soul forever hopeful. I would see a soul full of absolute trust that I would not, could not, give up on you. I felt ashamed of myself at these times when I clearly saw that light of strength shining in your eyes, and I knew that giving up was not an option.

It was at those times when we would end up in the hospital that I would see a child so much more worse off than you, a child who was definitely going to die that I would find myself feeling thankful that at least you had something that we could fight with pills, that at least you weren't facing something that was untreatable, something that, without doubt, was going to take your life, or so we thought at the time.

Hospitals were a big part of our lives. There are two hospital stays that stick out in my mind as reminding me of how lucky we were that pills could help you.

When you were in the children's hospital, when we were trying to find out why you kept turning blue, we were put in a room with a little boy who was about three years old. He had had a stroke shortly after birth. Seizures were a result of this and he sometimes had twenty seizures in an hour. As I sat next to your bed, I would hear the little boy cry out in pain. I watched as his grandmother gathered him in her arms and rocked him while singing him a lullaby in Spanish. She held him next to her body until she was convinced that his pain had passed. I found myself selfishly feeling both relief that your condition was not that bad and a pain deep in my soul for the suffering that I knew this family was experiencing. I felt my throat tightening and my eyes burning as I fought to keep my tears in check. I felt that I should have turned my head and not intruded on something so deeply private. I wish that more people could have been witness to this testimony of love. Maybe then they would start to realize that we parents of disabled children love our children as much as the parents of normally developing, healthy children love theirs, but we are much more aware that tomorrow is not guaranteed.

The other hospital stay that seems to most poignantly remind me of how thankful I should have been occurred during a stay at a local hospital. An African-American woman was there with her nine-month-old little girl. The little girl couldn't move. She had a degenerative neurological disorder that, the mother had been told, would take her life before she reached the age of one. This woman had already lost a son to this disorder and was now facing the loss of another child. I learned this as the woman and I got to know each other.

The love that this mother felt for her child was reflected in everything that she did. She gently sponge-bathed her, dressed her in beautiful pressed outfits, and outfitted her hair with bows and barrettes. When she talked to her little girl, her voice sounded almost like music, both soothing and hopeful. I watched as this girl's beautiful face lit up with love. She had one of the most beautiful faces that I had ever seen.

This woman never complained and, if one didn't look into her eyes, would have seemed a woman with a mountain of courage. I did look, though, and I saw a soul ravaged by pain. It was experiences like this that made me feel thankful that the imminence of your demise was not as near as this woman's child's. There was, for us, still hope that some therapy or operation or medicine would come along to save you. It was at those times, when modern medicine was providing us with little to no hope, that, with hope in tow, someone would enter our lives and offer us hope through observation or spiritualism.

The nurse at your first elementary school was a very religious person. She immediately took a liking to you and gave us a set of prayers to say twice a day for a year and a half, after which time, she said you would be healed. I knelt beside your bed every morning and night, head bowed, saying these prayers religiously (no pun intended), most times with tears running down my face. I needed to believe beyond belief that in a year and a half you would have the life that you deserved, free of illness. A year and a half went by, though, and ... nothing. Maybe I tried too hard. Maybe I didn't try hard enough. I found myself needing to find some justification for this, so I convinced myself that maybe I hadn't prayed hard enough, maybe I hadn't believed strongly enough. Surely I had done something wrong.

When people that we knew suggested "healers" whom they had heard were the "real thing," I put you in the car and took you to see them. I took you to a Catholic church the third Thursday of every month because the priest was said to have healing powers.

Daddy and I took you to a church where a "healer" was going to be. This particular trip was kind of funny. We always got to go to the head of the line because you were a child. Daddy and I brought you before this man. The man put his hand on your head and shouted out, "Speak, child, speak." You could have heard a pin drop. You looked at him with a quizzical look, probably wondering why he was yelling at you. Daddy and I were both holding our breath, waiting to see if you *would* speak. You didn't. If you had, I truly believe that both Daddy and I could have been knocked over with a feather.

In our search for miracles, when we were offered the opportunity to take you to Lourdes, we felt that we had no choice but to accept this gift, thinking it God's will. We felt that we had no choice but to give it a try. It seemed that on this trip, you did receive something, as your bad eyesight appeared to have been fixed. We did not discover this until shortly after we returned home from Lourdes.

When we got back from Lourdes, you would not keep your glasses on. Each time we put them on, you would pull them off and throw them on the floor. Then you started digging at your eyes, so we took you to see your ophthalmologist. Daddy held you down while the doctor examined you. He looked in one eye, said, "Huh!" He then looked at your chart. He looked in your other eye and said, "Huh!" He then looked at your chart again. He went back and looked in both of your eyes again. He said, "Huh!" Daddy finally asked if something was wrong. The doctor told him that, no, nothing was wrong. He said, "His vision is almost perfect. He is just very slightly nearsighted!" Your eyesight had been 20–400 prior to going to Lourdes. Daddy asked him if this happened very often and was told that it never happened.

This was not what I would have chosen to be "fixed," but I rationalized this by believing that you ... we ... had something else that we had to learn or achieve or teach by your continued suffering.

So when you were nine years old, when Grandma told us about a man called John of God, whom she had learned about on a news program, we decided to make the journey to Brazil to see if maybe he could heal you. After being told about this man, I went online and did some research. I also ordered a book about him. It seemed to me that miracles were indeed taking place down there, so we made plans to take you to see him. When modern medicine fails to effect a cure, and not just treat symptoms, people tend to become a whole lot more spiritual. I decided that if mankind couldn't provide a cure, maybe God could. I'm not sure how keen Daddy was on going, but I told him that I was going to go with or without him. If there was a chance that you could be cured by a higher being, if there truly is a higher being, I was willing to give it a try.

I guess that I was too naïve to know that this was something that I should have kept to myself. I was excited and hopeful, but I was to find out that this was one of those things that you shouldn't share with other people. I later found out that I had been thought a fool after telling people of our plans. I found out that those people that I had discussed John of God with had used this information to make both Daddy and I appear to be ridiculous religious zealots. They had used this information to try to mar Daddy's reputation. I felt so bad for Daddy. I didn't feel foolish, though, only angry.

So many people claim to believe in God but draw the line at extending that belief to miracles. It seems to me that you can't truly believe in one without believing in the other. It just doesn't make sense. It wasn't like I was going to be so trusting as to stop your medicines or medical treatments. I was going to give this a shot. I was going to dare to believe that God might bestow a miracle of healing on you, that God might decide that you had suffered enough and give you a shot at living a life free of disease. I was going to give you this opportunity, no matter what the gossipmongers had to say. They weren't living our, or your, life. Maybe if they had, they, too, might have been courageous enough to step out of their box and dare to dream of a miracle.

Daddy took care of everything. He arranged for us to get passports. He went and got our travel visas. He made the flight arrangements and arranged for us to be met at the airport with oxygen tanks for you. We were scheduled to arrive in Brazil on a Sunday and return home two weeks later. He went out and purchased everything that he thought that we might need while in Brazil so that you would not be inconvenienced. We were prepared for anything and everything!

This made us very popular with the people in our tour group as well as neighbors at the casa where we stayed.

We were met in Brasilia on Monday by Adrienne, one of our tour guides, and then taken by van to an exclusive resort to spend our first night in Brazil and give us the opportunity to get to know the other people in the group whom we would be spending the next two weeks with. There was a man in our group from Denver who knew one of the people who had been on the news special. He told us that the woman featured on the program was actually making progress after twenty years of having made no progress with regard to her paralysis. She and one of the cameramen had actually fallen in love!

We all piled back into the van the next day to begin our four-hour journey up the mountain to Abadiania. You thought that you were so big seated by the window of that van! You sat there, good as gold, taking everything in. Travelling always seemed to be in your blood. Maybe you were an adventurer in another life! When we finally reached our destination, we were given our room assignments and retreated to our rooms to rest and catch our breath.

It is really strange how things worked out. The couple in the room next to us, Bob and Mairead, had a little boy with seizures. His seizures seemed to be as bad as yours, except you handled the medicine well, while his seemed to make him awfully tired. He was beautiful, though, and sweet as can be. The four of us got along famously! Bob was a real smartass, and his wife was a comedian, so this helped to lighten the mood.

We hung out with Bob, Mairead, and Bobby when we weren't involved in activities with our group. Bob was hilarious! It was Bob who had wanted to make the journey to see John of God. Mairead had been the skeptic. I don't think that Bob was as strong a believer as he professed to be when he first arrived. Hoping and believing are two different things. I believe that everyone who visited that place had, at the very least, hope and were making their hardest effort to believe, but I think that actual belief only comes after experiencing something positive.

We went before John of God on Wednesday morning. You were prescribed "surgery," which was to occur later that afternoon, and the waterfall. Daddy was told to go sit in the meditation room as well as go to the crystal baths and the waterfall.

When I went before John of God, he reached out and took my hand and held it as he gave directions in Portuguese, which had to be translated for me. He had not done that with either you or Daddy. He must have recognized the despair, total exhaustion, and loss of hope that I was feeling over the way our lives were going. He must have sensed the constant struggle and the feeling that there was no visible light at the end of the tunnel. This was pretty evident, though, as no matter how hard I tried not to cry, I still had tears streaming down my face when I went before him. I was praying so hard that God would give us a break and fix what our lives had become. Daddy and I were exhausted, and I have no doubt that you also were. Our lives consisted of constant work, and watching you suffer valiantly day after day was taking its toll on all of us, but you always kept trying.

You were going from the time that you got up in the morning to the time you went to bed. You went to school, then saw up to three therapists a day, and then did discreet trials, sometimes keeping you up until ten at night You were so good about it. You were generally very patient and cooperative, even when I knew you were so very tired.

Daddy worked very long hours too. He worked at his primary job in the evenings and performed the duties that were his part of my business in the morning before going to work.

I was always the first one up and the last one to go to bed. I was generally up between three and four in the morning for years and didn't get to lay my head down on the pillow until around midnight. This was every day, every evening, every weekend. I went for five years without having a single day off and would not have taken any time off after that had we not gone in search of miracles. But I had decided that, come hell or high water, I was not going to miss an opportunity to procure a miracle for you if one was indeed awaiting us.

John of God told me to sit in the meditation room, just a few seats away from him. I remember sitting in the meditation room and suddenly feeling totally exhausted. I think that I kept falling asleep, as my head kept nodding forward, feeling too heavy to hold up. I was also prescribed crystal baths and the waterfall. We were all given herbs.

We all went to the waterfall later that day. We had to go in separate groups, the men and the women, so Daddy had to take you. The water was absolutely freezing! It took my breath away. I felt like I was going to hyperventilate! I have to say, though, that it was a sauna as compared to the baths in Lourdes! It wasn't so bad on subsequent trips to the waterfall, so it must have had something to do with my expectations. We were in a tropical environment, so I just didn't expect the water to be cold, and when it was, it probably just initially felt colder than it actually was. As I sat underneath the waterfall and the water rushed over my body, I opened my eyes and took in the area around the waterfall. I had this feeling like I was in a cocoon, like I was dreaming. And then I saw a blue butterfly flitter by my face. It really was a weird feeling. Maybe it was just hypothermia.

When we met up at the top of the trail, Daddy said that you had had a couple of quick seizures while at the waterfall. You were probably wondering whether we had finally lost our minds, putting you into frigid water again.

We then went back to our room to get dressed and go back before John of God for your surgery. The "surgery" was performed and we were instructed that you were not to leave our room for twenty-four hours. You were okay with this. You had your videos and books and two people to wait on you hand and foot, providing for your every need. What else could a little boy need? Except for the bed rail. We had not put the bed rail on your bed and you, always trusting that we would keep you safe, rolled over, book in hand, and fell to the floor. The look on your face was priceless! It was a "What the hell happened?" kind of look.

The day after we all went before John of God, Daddy told me an interesting story. He said that the night after seeing John of God earlier in the day, he had been trying to sleep and had awoken to the sound of the fan. Daddy has been deaf in his right ear since he was a baby due to viral meningitis. He would sleep with his left ear on the pillow so that he would not hear anything while he was sleeping. He thought that he must have been sleeping on the wrong ear. He turned over, but could still hear the fan. He then realized that he could hear out of his right ear! I found myself feeling envious, as it had been my idea to make this journey and yet I had not noticed any changes in myself or you.

On the third day there, we were walking back from our meeting with John of God when a woman hesitantly approached us. She said that she had seen us the day before but had not known whether she should approach us. She told us that she felt compelled to approach us that day because, she said, every time she walked by you, she got this strange sensation, felt the hair stand up on her arms, and got goose bumps all over. She said that she felt that you had been someone important in another life, someone who had been written about.

While we were there, we met the man with the astrocytoma who had been featured on the news special. He had received word that day per an MRI that the astrocytoma was gone. He had decided to marry a local woman, whom he had met on his numerous trips to Brasilia over the previous two years, and was making Brasilia his home.

When the weekend arrived and John of God went off to minister to people in other parts of the country, Gary and Adrienne took us down the mountain into Brasilia to visit some religious spots. Our first stop was at a prayer garden. We were told to follow the path to the middle and then back out, meditating all the while. I guess that I must really suck at meditation because I have never been able to be receptive to any life-altering revelations while trying to meditate. It kind of made me feel a further failure by not being able to do this.

We almost hated to leave when it came time to go. We had met so many kind people while we were there. The people who went there had basically been told by mainstream medicine that there was no hope or help for them, that they were never going to get better. But these people refused to believe that the medical professionals' word was the final word. I don't know if it was desperation or hope that led us all there. It was probably a combination of both of those things. I just know that I felt accepted there. I didn't feel like we were the "odd men out" for the first time in a long time. We weren't mistreated there, like we were in the "real" world. The people we met were open-minded, compassionate, and nonjudgmental. I didn't feel the need to offer up any explanations for anything while there and didn't find myself lying in wait for the next name-calling session. I felt hope there. I did not get for you what I had hoped to get and I found myself wondering why. I questioned why, if miracles do truly exist, you were not deemed worthy of one. That is an answer I am still waiting for.

They call this, I believe, a crisis of faith. I would like to say that I can no longer believe in an entity who would deny you the miracle of a clean bill of health and the ability to live a normal life, but I always found myself periodically begging and bartering with God. In my frustration, I found myself calling him names that even a drill sergeant would blush at hearing. I saw an episode of *House* where a nun said, "You cannot not believe in God and hate him at the same time," so I guess there is something in me, maybe just hope that there is some magnanimous being out there, who is on my side.

You Taught Me That We Can Only Truly Understand Anything by Actually Experiencing It, by Living and Breathing It

People always like to say that they understand what you are going through, but the truth is that no one can truly understand anything unless they themselves have gone through it. They can read books about something, watch a movie or television show, or listen to someone describe something, but they cannot truly understand what someone else is going through. This is because everyone experiences things differently. There are many factors involved in whatever someone is experiencing and those factors vary from person to person.

I know that people are trying to show kindness when they try to comfort you by saying that they understand what you are going through, but understanding cannot provide comfort. Time may possibly be the only thing that *can* provide comfort, but each of us has our own way of self-soothing and people need to be willing to be understanding of *that* fact. What works for one person may not necessarily work for another. We are, each of us, individuals and each have our own way of working through our pain.

I can remember thinking that saying that I understood what someone was going through was therapeutic for that person, but you showed me the truth where that is concerned. You taught me things that I could never have learned in a classroom, things that only you could teach me, things that could only be learned through experience. Experience is, and always will be, the most thorough and memorable teacher.

You Taught Me about Grace

You have been teaching me about grace since the day that you were born. You rarely complained about anything and endured most every situation with a strength of body and spirit rarely seen in this world. I used to think that it was because you didn't know any differently, that you thought the things that you were experiencing were experienced by everyone. I don't feel that way anymore.

I know that you tried to teach me by example, that we can get through anything if we just don't get lost in the discomfort, pain, attacks on our character, or any other things that are unpleasant in life if we just hold on to our beliefs and our sense of who we are. I saw you smile and laugh when you were feeling unwell, following the attack of a seizure on your body, or just because you were sick, and having been mistreated and called names by people who had no reason for that kind of behavior. I always called you "my little bumble" because you bounced back relatively quickly from anything that life threw your way.

I have to tell you, honey, that this is the one lesson that I have been unable to learn. I have tried to follow your example, but my love for you always seems to generate anger towards people, circumstances, the medical world, and any higher beings that might exist.

This is a hurdle that I cannot seem to get past. I have tried repeatedly and have almost made it, but then something else would happen and that hurdle only got higher, reaching heights I found myself unable to scale.

I apologize for having failed you in this aspect. It is not that you weren't an extraordinary teacher, it is just that the love that I felt for you incapacitated me when I saw how hard you tried, how valiantly you fought through things, and yet the powers that be stood in the way of your success. I watched you struggle, never giving up, and it angered me that you were not allowed to win when you were more deserving of winning than anyone that I have ever known. It is for this reason that grace has remained beyond my reach.

You Taught Me to Grow Up

All of the lessons that you taught me, made me truly grow up. I thought that I was already grown up when you came along, but as with most other beliefs that I have held, you showed me how wrong I was. You presented me with that rare opportunity to see the world through eyes other than my own. You both opened up and closed my world. I saw how cruel, as well as how kind, people can be. I learned that it is not the number of friends that you have but the quality and sincerity of those friends that matters most. I have learned what it feels like to be on the outside looking in, wondering why I am not allowed to be a part of the group. I learned how to be selfless, how to gladly put someone else's needs before my own. I learned to fight when something is worth fighting for. I understand that judgment of another human being should be based solely on the quality of their character and nothing else. I learned to be compassionate as well as tolerant.

I read back over your diary before I started writing this letter and was reminded of the extent of your suffering not only from your medical conditions but also, at the hands of the human race. I always thought that I had dealt with the pain associated with watching your little body and mind go through all the torment that it has. I now realize that I had only put those memories in storage. I had sent the pain into hibernation where it lay in wait to explode to the surface when I dared to let my guard down. I had stored it away in a place where I didn't have to deal with it right away because I had so many other things on my plate. There was just not enough time. Each time something happened, I had to take the attitude that we had again gotten through a terrible experience and I had to let it go. Dwelling on these experiences was of no value to anyone. I had to think about you and not me.

As I read your diary, though, I felt myself re-experiencing the gut-wrenching fear and grief that I had initially felt each time I had watched your little body beating itself up while I waited for your medicine to come to your rescue. With God as my witness, I would have switched places with you without a moment's hesitation if I could have prevented you from having to experience even one second of suffering, but we are not given that option.

Honey, I know that I overkissed, overhugged, and overloved you, and I suppose that I owe you an apology for being so needy. I, however, lived under a cloud of uncertainty where you were concerned and never knew which kiss, which hug, which touch, which "I love you" would be my last. I never knew if or when that seizure or bout of pneumonia would occur that would refuse to let you come back to me and leave me struggling to survive that proverbial Humpty Dumpty syndrome. I am not sure whether "all the king's horses or all the king's men" would ever be able to put me back together again should that happen but was always acutely aware that it was a very real possibility.

If I had never had you, I would be like the rest of them. I would only possess the ability to judge a book by its cover. I would not have been given the opportunity to see inside that book and read the thousands of pages contained between those covers. I would not have had the opportunity to rub elbows with a true hero. You gave me that. I would not have known the strength of the human spirit. You also gave me that. I stand humbled in the shadow of your greatness.

You were love incarnate, an angel brave enough to enter the human realm in a broken body. Your presence in my life has been the greatest gift that I could ever have received. I regret not always appreciating that gift, but having you by my side always made my life a life worth living. I, even knowing that your health condition was precarious at best, sometimes took your presence for granted, one of the mistakes that we as human beings seem to do, never having the strength to even consider the fact that life can be taken from us without a moment's notice. I think of all of the discrimination that you valiantly faced, the pain you endured on a daily basis, and the pain that caused you, Daddy, and me, but I can say without hesitation that I would not have missed having you for the world.

Thank you for choosing me to be your mother. Thank you for believing in me. Thank you, most of all, for loving me.

You are the love of my life. I can only hope that you know how desperately I love you. Always have, always will.

Love,

Mom

Epilogue

We recently lost our son, my husband and myself, and our hearts are broken. We believe that he would want the work he started on this earth to continue with regard to making the world a more hospitable place for the disabled, to make the world understand that the disabled want the same things that we all want. They want to be treated with dignity and not pitied. I do not believe that they pity themselves and do not welcome this particular emotion in their lives. Pity is an enabling emotion that serves no good purpose to either those who are its recipients or those people doling it out.

We received a letter from my sister following his death that, I think, is a fitting ending to his earthbound story.

> Could I erase your anguish, I would shake
> heaven and earth to do so,
> But I cannot ease your burden nor make sense of the moment.
> The anemic frailties of our human conditions.
> Were it possible to love or will another to
> health, surely it would have been so
> In this instance by adoring parents,
> Seldom equaled in their long, committed
> struggle to do so for their son—
> Or by any of we many family and friends
> Who were instantly and forever bewitched
> by this precious, lovely child.
> How elevated we all were by him gracing our lives.
> This sweet boy, too quickly grown into a young man—
> His entire life teaching us all by example,
> Too often called upon to fight the most difficult battles,

Yet undiminished in his capacity to love,
gentleness of heart and ability to laugh—
More a giggle paired with that sweet smile, empathy towards others
and endless determination of spirit, unjaded by the
insensitivities of smaller minds or lesser hearts.
There are no truer attributes of a hero.
Heroic as well, those who would dedicate their lives to
loving, guiding and nurturing such a relevant life.
I pray you strength to gather yourselves against
the difficulties of the days ahead,
That you will attend to the onerous task of
healing your own wounded spirits.
Joseph will continue to journey with you
throughout all the days of your lives.
He is intrinsic in your DNA.
It would be impossible to extract his profound
influences on your very beings,
For the memories the three of you created together have
left an indelible imprint on your hearts and souls.

About the Author

My husband and I reside in North Carolina and, until recently, lived there with our son, Joseph. We were an average family who, through our son Joseph, lived an extraordinary life. Together we faced situations where we were constantly having to confront people and professionals and fight for our son's rights to live in a world where he was the exception and not the rule.

Joseph was born with multiple medical problems, but he was a fighter right to the end. I believe that he came here knowing what he would face, but like any true hero, he faced these things with an amazing grace. He introduced us to the world of the disabled. I believe that he came here to teach us about that world and ultimately inform the world of the discrimination and cruelty faced by those people, who, through no fault of their own, are different than the general population.

An author named Taylor Caldwell wrote a book entitled *Bright Flows the River*, and there is a quote in it that, I think, fits Joseph perfectly. She wrote, "Bravery is more than courage, for it knows the terror it faces, but courage is only hope that the terror is less than it appears, so take it on."

He had diagnoses of Lennox-Gastaut syndrome, which is a seizure disorder resistant to medications, and autism. He had multiple seizures every day, and we had to watch his little body beat itself up until his medication could stop the seizure.

He went into status epilepticus numerous times. I would give him his rectal medication and, while I waited for the medicine to kick in, would kiss his little face, tell him that I loved him over and over again, and beg him to come back to me. When the seizure was finally over, he would put his little arm around my neck and give me a weak laugh, knowing that I needed the comfort that only he could give me. He would then vomit and go to sleep, going into what is referred to as a postictal period. When he awoke, he was the same happy boy that he always was, acting as if nothing of significance had happened.

It seemed that we could not leave the house without someone exacting cruelty on him in the form of derogatory statements, cruelty that was unwarranted but nevertheless something that we faced each time we ventured out into the world.

I do not think that people thought that he understood the cruel words thrown his way, but he understood everything. He rarely let any of these things get him down because he knew that he had parents who loved him unconditionally. I believe that this gave him the confidence to valiantly face the unconscionable treatment directed at him.

I have never met anyone with the amount of bravery and grace that my son had, except when coming into contact with other disabled individuals who have faced comparable treatment. Joseph had malice towards no one and, I believe, the gift of forgiveness, a gift common in the disabled. This is a strength of character that, should it be emulated by those nondisabled people, would make this world a better and more peaceful world to live in.

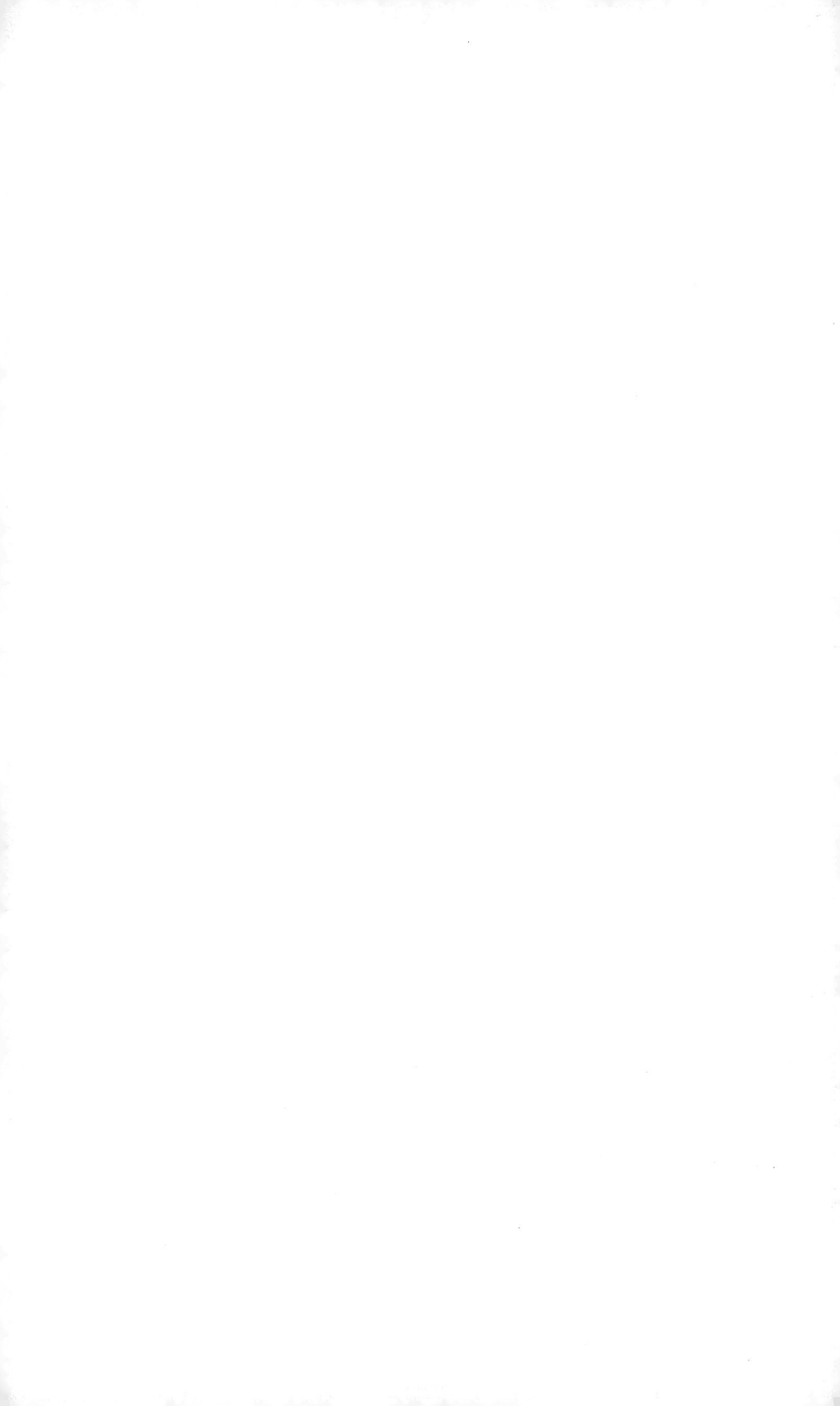

CPSIA information can be obtained
at www.ICGtesting.com
Printed in the USA
BVHW07s2119111018
529897BV00002B/479/P